Can't Hardly Breathe

By

Stormy Fanning

Can't Hardly Breathe

Chapter One

I sometimes wonder what I would have been if I hadn't become a nurse. I think we all wonder these things every so often. I really love being a nurse, though, and most days it seems to fit me pretty well.

Today, however, I am seriously questioning my choice. Nobody in nursing school ever mentioned that I might end up covered in dog poop and they skimmed over the part where I would have people swearing and swinging at me. They did teach me some mostly ineffective ways to 'de-escalate' the situation. I can't remember what they are right off hand- I'm too preoccupied with avoiding an elbow to the face.

This shift started out perfectly normal. They almost always do. A couple minor cases- some abdominal pain, a headache and a twisted knee. The weather was gray and cold, so nobody seemed to be out and about much. I was entertaining myself with the stack of magazines we had in a drawer for shifts like this.

Then, about 10 o'clock, the radio went off that the police needed an ambulance. The address was in a sketchier part of town, where several people were crammed in one house, even though none of them officially lived there. It was where people who wanted to disappear in a crowd went to disappear.

Since I was already contaminated, I decided to finish getting his clothes off before I cleaned myself up. We just cut the t-shirt off and threw it away then started working on getting his jeans and shoes off. His shoes were tied tight enough I couldn't just slide them off, but the laces were tied in knots and packed with dog poop. Just to be helpful, Trent kept trying to kick me as I was working on getting his shoes untied.

"Trent, knock it off!" Officer Hale said firmly. He pinned down Trent's leg for me, but Trent still kept kicking his foot side to side. "Knock it off, now!" Officer Hale repeated. "Don't you think you're in enough trouble already?"

"I didn't do nothin' wrong!" Trent replied, belligerently. "You ain't got nothin' on me. You're just a cop. You ain't nothin'. I got nothin'. You ain't gonna get me. This is just....this ain't.....just don't do nothin'." His rant lost steam as he seemed to forget what he was trying to say. We didn't have results on a blood alcohol level yet, but my guess was it was about 400. He was pretty tanked.

I finally got both shoes off and started to slide off his jeans. Trent suddenly became amused that a girl was undressing him.

"Hey baby, why you takin' my pants off?" he slurred as he smirked at me. I wanted to throw up. Did the falling-down-drunk covered in dog poop really think I was trying to come on to him? Sadly, yes he did.

“Trent, we have to get your dirty clothes off so we can wash you up,” I explained calmly. “We need to fix that cut on your arm.”

Trent looked down at his arms for a moment. “There ain’t no cut,” he replied bluntly.

“It’s on the underside of your arm,” I said, as I pointed to the spot on his left forearm that was covered in blood. He tried twisting his arm up so he could see it, but he couldn’t get it in the right position. He kept turning his arm side to side and then bending it up at the elbow, but never managed to get the angle right.

“There ain’t no cut,” he insisted. I took my gloved hand and touched the spot gently.

“Ow!” he yelped and jerked away.

“See, Trent, that is where the cut is,” I explained. He looked at me suspiciously, as if he thought I had just caused that injury. I wasn’t going to argue with him. I now had all his clothes off except his far-from-clean boxer shorts, and they were staying on, as far as I was concerned. I grabbed some washcloths and warm, soapy water and started washing him off, starting with the laceration on his arm.

It seems that dog poop in a laceration is not painful, but soap and water is. Trent howled and let loose a string of swear words, then swung at me with is other arm. Officer Hale grabbed the right arm and pinned it down, so Trent tried to hit me with his left elbow. Attacking the ER nurse right in front of the police officer is really a bad idea.

Apparently, Trent had enough alcohol on board, that didn't occur to him. I would have thought that much booze would numb any pain he was having. I guess he was at the level where he still had pain, but not much common sense.

I pinned Trent's left arm down by his wrist and finished washing up the arm. I put some gauze with disinfectant over the cut until the doctor could come in and suture it. Dr. Wallace was on today, and he hadn't even looked in the direction of this room yet. I'm sure he could hear and smell what was going on and he was waiting as long as he could to join the melee.

Every time I let go of Trent's arm, he tried to swing at me again, so Officer Hale put the hand cuffs back on him. That seemed to remind Trent that he was on his way to jail, and he calmed down and cooperated with the rest of the cleaning process.

Once I had Trent as clean as possible, I put all the dirty linens in the laundry hamper and bagged up Trent's shoes and jeans to go to the jail with him. Now I had to figure out how to get down the hall, covered in dog poop, without anyone seeing me. Then I had to peel off the dirty scrubs without smearing the poop around. It's a trick that most nurses have to learn at some point.

I peeked out the door and saw that the hall was clear right now. I scurried down the hall, turned the corner to the locker room, and nearly crashed into our CEO. What was he doing back here?

He took a step back and then sniffed and my face turned bright red. “I’m sorry, Mr. Albright,” I gasped. I looked at his crisp, navy suit and immaculate white shirt, hoping against hope I hadn’t managed to get any dog poop on him.

“What is on you, Allie?” he asked, with a concerned look on his face.

“It’s, um, we had a patient, that, um, had some…dog poop,” I stammered. I really wanted to give a good reason why I was covered in dog poop in the middle of the ER.

He smiled bemusedly. “I hope you’re headed in to change,” he said.

“Yes!” I replied emphatically.

“Well, I won’t keep you,” he said and gestured me past him to the locker room. I scurried through the door, carefully peeled off my dirty scrubs and bagged them up, then stood there in my skivvies as I scrubbed my arms, hands and face. Once I was certain I had all the poop washed off, I put on a pair of hospital issue scrubs. The hospital laundry doesn’t use fabric softener, since it can cause allergic skin reactions, so the hospital scrubs are scratchy and statickey. They are unisex sizing, so my options are being squeezed into a small or swimming in a medium. I went with swimming and just cinched up the drawstring pants as tight as I could.

I went back to the desk to find Dr. Wallace and let him know we were ready for him to suture. He nodded without enthusiasm and then sat there for a moment, gathering up the ambition to go in the room. Finally, he sighed and stood to his feet. 'Might as well get this over with' his expression said.

I didn't really want to go back in the room either, but we had to get Trent stitched up so we could send him on down the road. I followed Dr. Wallace in to the room, since I was sure I was going to have to help hold Trent down.

Trent was in the middle of some tirade directed at Officer Hale. He was quite sure his rights were being violated and he was not going to stand for it. Ironically, he was threatening to call the cops on them. Officer Hale didn't bother trying to explain that he *was* the cops.

"Hello, I'm Dr. Wallace and I need to look at your arm," he introduced himself. Trent looked at him for a long moment, trying to process what he had said.

"All right, doc, fix me up," he finally said. "Give me some of the good stuff."

"We'll use lidocaine to numb the area," Dr. Wallace explained. Trent had a colorful response to that.

"I want some good stuff!" he demanded. "I want some morphine up in there!"

Dr. Wallace paused for a moment. There were a few things wrong with Trent's demand. Morphine doesn't have any local anesthetic properties. Injecting morphine in the cut wasn't going to do anything. And morphine is a bit of overkill for a simple laceration. Plus, giving narcotics to a guy who is already loaded up on alcohol is a bad idea. Basically, morphine was out of the question. Now to explain that to Trenton. Dr. Wallace wasn't very patient, even under the best circumstances, so this could be interesting.

"Morphine isn't the indicated drug," Dr. Wallace started to explain.

"Bull!" Trent yelled at him. "I want some morphine! Give me some morphine now or I'm not gonna do it!" He sprinkled his demands with plenty of expletives. Dr. Wallace didn't care much for swearing, and what little patience he had vanished quickly.

"No," he said bluntly. "You're not getting morphine. No more swearing either. I'm sewing up your arm and you're going to jail." He stared at Trent, with his arms crossed across his barrel chest. Trent stared back for a minute, but he must have realized he was going to lose this battle.

"Fine," he muttered under his breath as he let his head fall back on the gurney. Officer Hale and I held the arm in place while Dr. Wallace made short work of closing up the laceration. He walked out of the room, tossing an order over his shoulder for me to give a tetanus shot to Trent before he left.

Trent didn't care for needles, it would seem. Well, medical needles anyways. He had several tattoos, so he had to tolerate some needles. But the mention of a shot got him all wound up again.

"I don't do shots. No way. Uh uh. Nope. Don't do it." He spouted off a half dozen different phrases to indicate he didn't want the shot. Technically, a patient has the right to refuse treatment. However, patients who are under the influence of alcohol or drugs are not in a clear frame of mind, so they aren't in a condition to make that decision.

I went and got the tetanus vial and the syringe and needle. I got back to the room and Trent was still babbling on and insisting he didn't want a shot. I stood so I was out of his line of vision and drew up the serum. Once I had it ready, I hid it down by my side.

"Trent, I just need to look at your arm," I said, pleasantly. "I'm just going to look at this spot right here." I gently squeezed his left deltoid to show him what I was looking at.

"Don't give me no shot," he insisted.

"I'm not going to give the shot yet, I'm just going to look at your arm," I said as I continued to squeeze the deltoid rhythmically and swabbed it with an alcohol pad. Trent was facing away from me, talking to Officer Hale about how much he hated shots. Still squeezing, I stuck the needle in and injected the serum. Trent didn't even notice. I rubbed his deltoid gently to work the injection in to the muscle.

"Ok, we're all done," I said cheerfully. I was pretty good at shots, so I had been sure I could get away with that.

Technically, I didn't lie to Trent. I told him I was going to look at his arm first. It just so happens I didn't need to look at it for very long.

Trent looked at me perplexed. Perhaps he thought he had won the argument and he wasn't going to get the shot. I was just ready to get him moved on out of the ER before we had any more excitement.

Officer Hale and his partner loaded up the now clean Trenton Queen and drove away. The ambulance had left long ago, and was probably back at the station, trying to clean out all the dog poop. Which was what I got to do in the room now.

After I got the room back to its original condition, I glanced at the clock and realized it was lunchtime. I didn't have much of an appetite yet, though, so I told the other nurse to go first. I could still catch a whiff of dog poop every so often. I even went back to the bathroom to make sure there wasn't any in my hair, but I didn't see any. Maybe the smell was just lodged in my nose. I couldn't wait to get home and take a hot, soapy shower.

Sandy, the front desk clerk on today, walked up to the nurses' station from her desk at the front. Sandy was slender and petite with sandy blond hair. She was very soft-spoken, which could be a problem sometimes in the hectic ER environment. But she was really nice and did a great job. We just had to ask her to repeat herself every so often.

"I have a lady in triage," Sandy said to me. She could never bring herself to just call out 'Triage' from the desk like the other clerks did. Maybe all the extra walking she did was what kept her so slender. I looked past her to the front desk, where a middle aged woman was sitting. She was slumped in the chair with her head in her hands. She was wearing dark glasses, and probably not because she thought she was cool. I had seen this look before.

I walked up to the desk and said softly, “How can we help you?” I was pretty sure she was here with a migraine headache and would be sensitive to noise as well as light.

“I have a migraine,” she said, tensely. “I haven’t had one in a really long time and I’m out of my pills.”

I asked her which migraine medication she took and she told me. She said they worked really well for her, but she forgot to refill her prescription after she took the last one. She hadn’t gotten a headache in over three months, but she was under a lot of stress this week and the pain had started this morning. It finally got bad enough she knew she wasn’t going to be able to fix it with ibuprofen. Unfortunately, her prescription had expired, since they’re only good for a year. Her doctor’s office couldn’t get her an appointment for three more days so the ER was her last resort.

Sandy completed the necessary check in paperwork as quickly as possible and then brought the patient, Marian Redmond, down the hall to a room. I followed her in the room, but didn’t turn on the light. I got her vital signs quickly and asked a few key questions.

"I hardly ever get headaches anymore," she explained. "This week has just been rough. My mom fell and broke her arm, so I'm trying to help her out as well as take care of my family too." That would be stressful. I kept my assessment brief, the sooner she could get a dose of medication the better.

I stepped out to let Dr. Wallace know about Marian. Then I got two small ice packs and brought them back in the room.

"Here's some ice packs," I told her as I wrapped them in a cloth.

"What are those for?" she asked.

"You put them on your forehead and the back of your neck," I told her. "It helps with the throbbing."

I carefully placed the pack on her neck and she leaned back on the gurney. I placed the other one across her forehead. I told her the doctor would be in soon, and pulled the curtain to block the light from the hall.

Dr. Wallace went in to see her briefly and then came out and gave me the order for the migraine medication. I got the pill and a glass of water to take back into the room.

"Marian, I have your medication," I said softly as I entered the room. She sat up and took the pill and swallowed it.

"That ice pack really helps," she said, sounding surprised. "I wonder why?"

"The cold makes the blood vessels in the brain constrict down," I explained. "It also works for hangovers," I added, laughing.

Marian smiled at that. "I don't have to worry about those anymore," she said. "But it definitely takes the edge off a migraine."

"Do you need a warm blanket to offset the ice pack?" I asked her. The ice helped the throbbing headache but tended to cool them down all over.

"No, thank you," she replied. "I think I'm going through the change. I'm always hot. This ice feels wonderful."

I told her I would check back in a bit to see if the meds were helping and gave her the call light. I went back to the desk to chart everything. Linda, the other nurse on duty, came back from lunch and told me I should go eat now. I filled her in on Marian and headed to the break room to eat.

My lunch today was leftover Chinese takeout from a few days ago. Chinese is great as leftovers. It doesn't go bad for days, even weeks. Must be all the chemicals they put in it. I warmed it up in the microwave and poured a glass of iced tea to go with it. Linda loved iced tea and always made a gallon of it to keep in the fridge when she was working. I liked iced tea, too, but it was better when it was already made and I didn't have to go to any trouble.

I ate my lo mein and checked my cell phone for messages. My dad had had a heart attack a few months ago, and ended up having open heart surgery. Since he had gone home, my mom kept in pretty frequent contact with me. They had a home health nurse, but mom seemed to prefer calling me. That was okay with me, I liked being kept up on how dad was doing. They lived in a small town about 45 miles away, so I couldn't just hop over there anytime. Dad had had some complications after surgery and I was still a little nervous about him. He was doing great, but I was a champion worrier.

All I had was a text message from my little sister, Shelby, complaining about the weather. Winter was definitely headed our way. I didn't care for the cold, but I loved to play in the snow. We weren't going to get snow for a few more weeks at least, though, so we just had to suffer through the cold. I sent a text back telling her to hang in there and daydream of powder, then stashed my phone back in my locker.

I headed back to the nurses' station to see how my patient was doing. Linda reported that Marian was now sound asleep, so she had decided to just leave her alone. Marian would probably appreciate the nap, I imagine she hadn't been sleeping well. Stress has a way of doing that to you.

Nothing else seemed to be going on, so I grabbed a seat. This weather wasn't doing much for my motivation level.

"So, Allie," Linda said, then paused. That meant she had something to ask me and it was usually about my dating life. She wasn't being nosy or gossipy, she was just very concerned that I was never going to get married and have kids. Maybe my mom was paying her on the sly to pester me about my single status.

"Yes, Linda," I replied with a smile. She knew I could see right through her.

"Met anyone interesting lately?" she asked.

"Well, I was in the grocery store last week and there was a guy in there," I told her. "He seemed interesting."

"Really?" she asked. "What's his name?"

"Oh, I didn't get his name," I said.

"Why not?" she asked. I was having fun with this, but I'm a terrible liar, so I wasn't going to be able to keep it up much longer.

"He didn't seem to like it when other people talked to him," I told her. "He was having a heated argument with his invisible friend and he didn't want to be interrupted."

Linda just shook her head at me and tried to hide her smile. "Allie, Allie, Allie," she said. "We need to find you a man."

I never knew what to say to comments like that. I knew Linda meant well, so I just shrugged it off.

"What we really need to do," she continued, "is knock that Jake upside the head so he realizes he should ask you out."

Eek. Now the conversation got uncomfortable. Jake was a paramedic on the local fire department, so our paths crossed fairly frequently with work. Jake was also incredibly good-looking and the cause of drooling in women from eighteen to eighty. I certainly wasn't immune to his good looks and warm hearted charm, but I was pretty sure that Jake flirted with most of the women he met. I wasn't going to delude myself that he was interested in dating me.

Besides, I wouldn't really want to be dating the guy that everyone drooled over. Too much competition. Most of our conversations involved work or medical drama, so who's to say if we were even that compatible. It takes more than striking blue eyes and dimples a mile deep to make a relationship.

Although the blue eyes and killer smile certainly didn't hurt!

Chapter 2

I was lying on the beach, feeling the warm sun on my face. My toes were curled in the sand and I could hear the gentle splashing of the waves lapping on the beach. I could hear a mariachi band playing in the distance, some song I had never heard before. It was an upbeat melody but one of the players was way off. He was making a shrill chirping noise that wasn't even in tempo with the rest of the band. And it kept getting louder.

I finally woke up enough to realize the shrill chirping noise was my alarm clock and I was nowhere near a beach. I hit the alarm and dragged myself out of bed. Maybe I needed to take a vacation. Of course, I didn't have anyone to take a tropical vacation with me and I imagine even the nicest beach gets lonely and boring by yourself.

I sighed and headed to the kitchen to make some toast for breakfast. One more shift and then I had a few days off. After yesterday's adventure, I didn't have much enthusiasm for one more shift, but I would be a little perkier once I got some coffee in me. I wasn't ambitious enough to get up early and make coffee at home before I left for work. I headed for the coffee pot in the break room as soon as I got to work, though. Caffeine was my addiction, and I had no interest in a twelve step program. My co-workers were happy to enable me, because me without caffeine was not a pretty picture.

I picked out a brightly colored set of scrubs, trying to channel the feeling of a tropical resort. I could hear the rain against the window, so I knew the actual weather was very un-tropical. But I could always pretend.

I had to put a heavy coat and gloves over my tropical outfit, though. This time of year the rain could quickly turn to snow, and it was best to be prepared. My imagination might entertain me, but it wouldn't keep me warm.

I got to work and stashed my stuff in my locker. I found my coffee cup in the cupboard and filled it with steaming hot coffee. I took the first sip and sighed happily. That was much better. I walked up to the nurses' desk to see how the night had gone.

The night shift crew were sitting there, bleary-eyed. I had worked night shifts for a while, and 7 a.m. was a rough time. In fact, the entire 4 a.m. to 7 a.m. stretch was a challenge.

"How was the night?" I asked.

"Horrible," replied Roger. "Long. We've only had three patients all night."

That would explain the bleary eyes. It's hard enough to keep awake when there's stuff to do. Sitting in a chair makes it nearly impossible. The bad weather was keeping people indoors, so we were less busy than usual.

"Well, if you're here, I'm going to go home," Roger said. "Hope your day is busier than the night was."

I did too. I didn't care for days that dragged on forever. Of course, I didn't really want to repeat yesterday's debacle again, but a steady stream of not-drunk patients would make the day go by quickly.

I really missed my pal, Lacey. She had been a nursing assistant, or CNA, in the ER up until last spring, when she graduated from nursing school. She was now doing her six month stretch working on the medical floor before she could train to the ER. I knew it was important for her to get a good, solid orientation to nursing. But I really missed working with her because she was a lot of fun. A shift with her flew by whether it was busy or not. She had two more months before she transferred to the ER and I couldn't wait.

I was just finishing my coffee when the ambulance radio went off. An eighty-three-year-old had fallen at Rosewood Court, an assisted living facility in town. She was complaining of hip pain, which is never a good sign. I walked in to the 'bones and bruises' room and turned up the thermostat. One thing I've learned about the octogenarian set is that they are always cold.

Dr. Robbins was on today, so that helped. Dr. Robbins had been an ER doctor for thirty years and he was pretty good at it. He was laid back, which helped keep stress levels down, but he also had a sense of humor. He was my favorite doctor to work with, that was for sure.

The other nurse today was Jesse, and he was not my favorite nurse to work with. He was incredibly lazy and always tried to get out of taking patients. It was irritating but I was used to it.

The radio crackled with the crew calling report. The EMT calling in was Kent, who was partners with Jake. My heart fluttered for a moment when I realized Jake would be coming in to the ER in just a few minutes. I sternly reminded myself that it was nothing more than work and went to the radio to take report.

Mrs. Gertrude Williams had gotten tripped up on a throw rug in her apartment and gone tumbling. She was complaining of right hip pain and she kept saying she was very worried that it was broken. The EMTs had carefully packed her up and brought her in to the ER to get checked out.

Gertrude was a little bit of a thing, with her white hair carefully coiffed and her rose-colored lipstick perfectly drawn on. She was wearing a silk blouse with dress slacks, complete with an earring and necklace ensemble. She was quite distraught, and kept saying over and over that she was worried her hip was broken. It was her right hip that she was concerned about. She did have pain to that hip but no other telltale signs like shortening or rotation of the leg. The first step was to get an x-ray.

I went through the necessary health history questions while we waited for the x-ray tech. Gertrude had just moved here a few months ago, when her husband passed away, because her kids were here. She had never been seen in our hospital before, so we didn't have any information on her. I had gotten through medications and allergies when the x-ray tech arrived to take her for her x-ray. I would finish the rest when she got back.

The x-ray didn't take long, and after the x-ray tech wheeled Gertrude's gurney back in to the room, he stopped off at the desk.

"Uh, doc, you might want to look at that one," he said with an amused look on his face. I was guessing it wasn't broken, since that wouldn't be amusing. I looked over Dr. Robbins' shoulder as he pulled up the digital images. There, staring back at us, were two artificial hips. Well, at least we knew they weren't broken! Since I hadn't gotten to the surgical history section yet, she hadn't had a chance to tell me she had had hip surgery.

Dr. Robbins walked in to the room to ask Gertrude about it and I followed along.

"Mrs. Williams, you have had a hip replacement on both hips," he said to her, and paused for her reaction.

"Oh, I know," she said. "I broke that right one just six months ago. That's why I was so worried it was broken again."

Dr. Robbins tried to hide his amusement. Obviously, her orthopedic surgeon hadn't communicated clearly what they had done. Or Gertrude just didn't understand it when he explained it.

"Mrs. Williams, that hip is made of titanium," Dr. Robbins said patiently. "You could jump out of an airplane and it wouldn't break."

"Really?" she said, sounding surprised. "I didn't realize that." She pondered that for a moment. "Are you sure about that?" she asked Dr. Robbins.

He finally lost the battle and actually laughed. "Yes, I am sure," he told her. "You might be able to break everything else on you, but you don't have to worry about breaking your hip ever again."

"Well, why does it hurt then?" she wanted to know.

"You can still bruise it," Dr. Robbins explained. "It may even be tender from your surgery still. We can give you some pain medicine to help for a few days after this fall. It should feel better within a week."

Gertrude looked relieved. I'm sure, after two hip replacements, she was glad she didn't have to go through hip surgery again. Dr. Robbins told her we would give her some ibuprofen for the pain and then see how she did walking before we sent her home.

I gave the medication and told Gertrude I would be back in twenty minutes to see if her pain was better. I walked back out to the desk, where Jake and Kent were standing. I had said 'Hi' briefly as they brought in the patient, but then I had been focused on taking care of her while they were writing up the ambulance report.

"So, her hip isn't broken, huh?" Jake said with a wry smile.

“No, her titanium hip is completely intact,” I laughed. “Which is good. Poor thing was worried for no reason.”

“Well, I’m glad she’s ok,” Kent said. “She was so polite. She even tried to offer us a snack.”

“Why was she so dressed up this early in the morning?” I asked.

“The staff said she always is,” Kent replied. “She moved here from the south, and she was raised to ‘always look a lady’, as she likes to say. They said they’ve never seen her without her hair and makeup done.”

I couldn’t relate to that. Today, my hair was ‘done’ because it was up in a ponytail and I didn’t have any stray pieces coming loose. I had some eyeliner and mascara on, but I didn’t even own a lipstick. I guess it was a good thing I didn’t live in the south.

“How’s your dad doing?” Jake asked me. When my dad had been in the hospital, Jake had been really good at listening to me vent when I got overwhelmed with everything. He still asked me about him whenever he saw me.

“Good,” I replied. “He even gave up bacon, except for on Sunday morning. He’s determined that he will never end up in the hospital again.”

“Well, that’s a good attitude to have,” Jake said. “If more people were like him, we might not have a job.” He smiled at me, teasingly. We both knew we would still have jobs. But we did see a lot of repeat customers and if more of them determined they were going to do everything they could to prevent getting sick again, we certainly wouldn't be as busy.

"Well, he's stubborn enough to make it work," I said. I didn't mind my dad's determination to stay healthy from now on. It gave me one less thing to worry about.

"I'm glad he's doing ok," Jake said, resting his hand on the back of my shoulder. His hand was warm and strong and incredibly distracting.

"Thanks," I replied, unable to think of anything else to say. I just smiled into his crystal blue eyes.

"We better get back to the station," he said. Did I hear a tinge of regret in his voice? No, just wishful thinking on my part, I'm sure. They said good-bye, Jake took his strong, warm hand off my shoulder and they walked out the door.

I went back to check on Gertrude, who was feeling much better. Now that she wasn't worried her hip was broken, she did a fine job of sitting up, standing, and even walking. Her daughter had arrived about ten minutes ago, and they both felt that Gertrude would be ok if she went back to her apartment. There was a staff nurse at Rosewood Court that could check in on her.

I helped Gertrude out to her daughter's car and wished her luck. She thanked me and they headed on their way. Dr. Robbins was sitting at the desk, still chuckling to himself. This job was certainly amusing some days.

Tracy was the front desk clerk on for the day, and I heard her call out 'Triage', so I headed up to the front. A heavyset woman in her twenties was sitting at the desk, looking a little pale, and holding a barf bag. As I walked up to ask how we could help her, she cried out and doubled over, clutching her abdomen. I was going to guess abdominal pain, nausea and vomiting and possibly diarrhea. We didn't need to drag this out. Tracy got the necessary information to get her checked in and I brought her down the hall to a room.

Her name was Kaeley Feinstein and she was twenty-six years old. She said the pain had started about four hours ago, but it was getting worse. She said it would come and go, like a really sharp cramp. She had been nauseous but hadn't thrown up much because she hadn't eaten anything. We went through the usual summary-medications, allergies, health history and surgeries. She said she didn't know when her last period was because her cycle was irregular. She had been diagnosed with polycystic ovarian syndrome, or PCOS a couple years ago.

She was a little abrupt when she was answering my questions, as if she were irritated that I was asking them. I reminded myself that she didn't feel well and I shouldn't take it personally. I had to ask all these questions to help figure out what was wrong, I wasn't doing it just to try her patience. I told her I would let the doctor know she was here and that when she needed to go to the bathroom, we would get a urine sample.

"Good luck with that," she said sharply. "I haven't drank anything all day."

I didn't really know what to say to that, so I didn't say anything. I went out to the desk and let Dr. Robbins know her situation. He went in to talk to her briefly and came back out to give me the orders. He wanted to place an IV and draw some blood as well as get an x-ray of her abdomen.

Since she was of child-bearing age, our policy required that we check a pregnancy test before we took an x-ray. That was part of the reason we collected a urine specimen. I went in to start the IV and explain to her that we needed a urine sample, even if it was a small amount.

"I don't have to pee," she snapped. "And I can't get pregnant, I have PCOS, remember?"

"Well, we have to be 100% sure," I explained to her. "Are you sexually active?"

She snorted and said, "It's been a while."

Since abstinence was a 100% effective form of birth control, if a female wasn't sexually active, we could consider that an 'all clear' for pregnancy. Of course, sometimes the person wasn't totally honest with us.

"We would rather be safe than sorry," I started to say, when she doubled over and clutched her stomach again.

After groaning for about a minute, she finally sat back up and glared at me. "I am sick!" she yelled. "Why don't you figure out what's wrong with me and stop bugging me about being pregnant? I am NOT pregnant!"

I went back out to the desk to talk to Dr. Robbins about this. He was hesitant as well to do the x-ray without a pregnancy test. Since women with PCOS believe they can't get pregnant, they often didn't use any form of birth control. She didn't necessarily *look* pregnant, but she was pretty round all over, so it was hard to determine.

Dr. Robbins went in to explain to her the risks of doing the x-ray without checking for pregnancy first. She cut him off quickly by insisting, "I haven't had sex since last year." It was now the end of October, so that would put her well past nine months since she last had sex. She was adamant that she couldn't give us a urine sample because she was too dehydrated and she just wanted the x-ray taken now. Dr. Robbins gave the ok for that, so we called x-ray.

She was looking pretty rough, kind of clammy and pale. Dr Robbins gave me an order to give some anti-nausea medication and some morphine while we waited. She didn't say anything while I gave the meds, but did double over in pain again. I didn't think she was faking the pain, that was for sure. She was obviously miserable, we just needed to find out why.

The x-ray tech came shortly and wheeled to the x-ray department. I caught up my charting while she was gone and made a quick bathroom break. Jesse had a couple other minor patients in, and I'm sure he was irritated that he was having to get up and work. That's ok, it was good for him.

The x-ray tech brought Kaeley back and put her back in her room. He walked back up to the desk looking pale, with his eyes wide.

"Uh, doc, you better look at that one," he said, and there was no amusement in his voice. Dr. Robbins pulled the digital image up on the computer and we all just stared at it for a minute. There, curled up in her abdomen, was a tiny little human, with its head wedged down between her pelvic bones. Kaeley was not only pregnant, she was in labor.

We all looked at each other, stunned, for a moment. How could she be pregnant if she hadn't had sex since last December? Dr. Robbins walked back in the room to ask her.

"Kaeley, you said you haven't had sex since last December," he said and then paused.

She looked sheepish and said, "Well, maybe January. I don't remember." That would make a little more sense. In fact, that would be about perfect timing to be full-term right now.

"Kaeley, you're pregnant," Dr. Robbins said carefully. "Your abdominal pain is actually labor."

She just sat there, stunned. She blinked a couple times and then just kept staring at him. I was worried she had slipped into a catatonic state when she suddenly doubled over in pain again.

I wanted to tell her to breathe through the contraction, but I knew she hadn't taken Lamaze classes. We waited for a minute for her contraction to subside. She finally looked back up at me and said, "I guess I did have to pee. I just wet the bed."

I met Dr. Robbins eye over the top of her head and we both were thinking the same thing. Kaeley didn't wet the bed, her water just broke. Technically, the baby could still take hours to come out, but we didn't want to take that chance. We didn't like delivering babies in the ER when we had a perfectly nice labor and delivery unit just down the hall.

"I'll call the OB doc," Dr. Robbins said as he walked out the door. I knew he was also going to have Tracy call the labor unit and tell them we would be bringing them a patient shortly.

I turned to Kaeley, who was crying, her face a mix of pain and fear. This was a lot to process all at once, and she didn't have much time to mull it over, since she was in active labor.

"Kaeley, is there someone we can call?" I asked. It didn't sound like the baby-daddy was in the picture but she must have a family member or friend to come sit with her during labor.

She shook her head, still crying. "My mom will kill me if she finds out about this," she said, her voice breaking.

"Well, you could call a friend, maybe," I suggested. She just shook her head again.

"I don't want anyone to know about this," she sobbed. I made a mental note to let the labor nurse know that Kaeley would need some information and counseling on what her options were and what resources were available to her. This was a terrible time to have to decide if you wanted to keep your baby or give it up for adoption.

I walked over and put my arm around her shoulders. This whole situation just broke my heart and I didn't know what to do. She leaned against me, still crying, then cried out and doubled over in pain again.

I hadn't been looking at the clock, but those last two contractions weren't very far apart. We needed to get her to the labor room, and the sooner the better.

I told Kaeley I would be right back and went out to see if everything was in place for us to transfer. Dr. Robbins had just gotten off the phone with Dr. Deitz, who was the OB on call for the day.

"He's headed in right now," Dr. Robbins told me.

"And the labor nurse is ready," Tracy chimed in. That was the green light I needed. I grabbed a wheelchair, placed some clean towels down to absorb the amniotic fluid and went back in Kaeley's room. She was now standing up and her pants were soaking wet, as well as the linens on the bed.

"Have a seat, Kaeley, and we'll get you to the labor unit," I said, gesturing to the chair. She walked over and started to sit, then stood back up with a funny look on her face.

“I can’t sit down,” she said. “It feels like something is in the way in there.”

My heart skipped a beat. That baby was coming fast, and I didn’t want to be in the catcher’s positions. I stripped the wet linens off the gurney, tossed them on the floor and took the dry linens out of the wheelchair and spread them on the gurney.

“Here, lay back down on the cart,” I told her. She got back on the cart with some difficulty. She still had pants on, so I couldn’t see if the baby’s head was crowning, but that was just as well. I was nervous enough as it was.

I covered her with a blanket and we headed down the hall. I was praying fervently as I pushed the gurney as quickly as I could without breaking into a run. I had gone through all the training for a precipitous delivery, but I didn’t want to have to use it. Newborns were so tiny and frail, I was scared of hurting them. Plus, they came out with extra stuff and I couldn’t exactly remember what I was supposed to do with all of it.

We wheeled in to the labor unit and Lori, the labor nurse, was standing in the hall. She pointed me into the first room and I wheeled the cart in. The room was already set up for a delivery with all the equipment in place. They even had a bassinet and baby warmer in the corner already. They were prepared and it was a good thing.

Lori started to ask Kaeley to stand up and walk to the labor table. I interrupted and told Lori that Kaeley could ‘feel something in there’, and a look of understanding dawned on her face. We slid Kaeley over to the labor table and pulled her bottoms off. Lori was ready to do a cervix check, but instead there was the top of a little head showing. Even I knew that meant we had a baby coming in short order.

"The baby is crowning," Lori said to Kaeley, who had the most terrified look on her face. I guess I had better bring Lori up to speed.

"Lori, Kaeley didn't know she was pregnant," I started out. "So she hasn't been through any prenatal care." Basically, that was the polite way of telling Lori that Kaeley didn't know what 'crowning' meant.

Lori looked at me, dumbfounded. "Um, Tracy didn't mention that on the phone," she said. "Does Dr. Deitz know that?"

"I think so," I replied. "Dr. Robbins talked to him."

Lori looked back at Kaeley and put a hand on her shoulder. "Honey, I know you must be freaking out," she said. Kaeley nodded vigorously. " We'll get you through it," Lori reassured her. "I'll be with you the whole time."

Kaeley looked a little relieved, but still terrified. I wanted to stick around and see how the rest of the labor went, but I knew I better get back to the ER. I gave Lori the rest of the information I had for report, but it was brief.

"Good luck, Kaeley," I said as I pushed the cart out the door.

She started to say something but another contraction started. I could see Dr. Deitz rushing down the hall, pulling his jacket off as he walked. I figured I had better just get out of the way, so I took my cart and headed back to the ER.

As I walked back down the hall, I tried to imagine what Kaeley would be going through right now. The idea of having a baby pretty much terrified me to start with. Everyone liked to tease me about my biological clock ticking, but so far, I hadn't heard it. I thought kids were a lot of fun, but also a lot of responsibility, and I wasn't sure I was ready for that. I wasn't married, so it wasn't an issue, anyways. Maybe I would worry about it more if I was.

But with the way my dating life was going, I wasn't going to have to worry about marriage or kids for a long time.

Chapter 3

I decided to call my parents and check in. We had always had a good relationship, close but not too close, but since my dad's surgery, I liked to check in a little more frequently. It was nice to talk to them anyway.

My dad answered, which surprised me, because my mom was usually the one who answered the phone. Dad would just sit there, listening to it ring and looking at mom expectantly, wondering why she wasn't answering it.

"Hi dad," I said. "How's it going?"

"Good," he replied. He was a man of few words, so that was going to be the extent of the conversation. Maybe that was why mom usually answered the phone

"Where's mom?"I asked.

Dad hesitated for just a moment before he replied, "She's laying down for a bit."

Something about the way he said that got my spidey senses humming. "What's wrong?" I asked sharply.

"Well," he started and then took a breath, and sighed. "She's been tired lately." He paused for a long moment, then continued, "I've been a little worried about her, actually."

"What?" I cried. "Why? What's wrong with her?"

"I dunno for sure," he said. "She's just pale and she wears out easy. She doesn't eat like she should and she just doesn't look so good."

"Dad, why didn't you tell me?!" I said, anxious and exasperated all at once.

"Well, I didn't want to worry you none," he said, in his usual calm manner. "Don't tell your mom I said she doesn't look good, either. She'll get mad at me."

I had to laugh at that. Mom wouldn't get mad over that comment, she would understand what he meant by it. He liked to make it sound like she was always getting mad at him. They actually got along pretty well, most of the time.

"Oh, here she is," he said and then I heard him say, "Betty, Allison is on the phone."

After a moment, I heard my mom say, "Hello, Allison." I strained to hear anything wrong in her voice, which was ridiculous, and I realized that, but I did it anyway.

"Hi mom," I said. "How are you feeling?" I decided to try the polite route first.

"Oh, I'm fine, honey," she replied pleasantly. "How are you?"

I didn't have much for patience anyway, so I cut right to the chase. "Mom, Dad says you've been tired a lot lately."

"Oh, a little," she hedged. "I'm not as young as I used to be," she laughed softly.

It was hard to argue with my mom that she really didn't feel good when she was insisting she was fine and I wasn't there to see her. I didn't want to start an argument between her and dad by telling her that he was worried about her.

"How long has this been going on?" I asked her. I was a natural born worrier, so I was trying to keep calm and not jump to conclusions, but I still had a bad feeling in my stomach.

"Well," she said and paused for a long moment. "I guess it's been over a month now." She sounded a little surprised. "I didn't realize it had been that long, but I started feeling tough back in September, right after the county fair got done."

"Besides being tired, are you having any other problems?" I asked.

"My stomach has been upset a lot," she said. "I don't seem to be able to eat much and that's probably why I'm tired." She sounded calm and matter-of-fact, so I knew she wasn't yet concerned enough to go to the doctor. But I would sleep a lot easier if she got checked out, so I was going to try to convince her to go.

"Mom, don't you think you should check in with Dr. Cullard?" I asked gently. "It's got to be time for a check-up anyway."

"Well, it's actually been a couple years since I went in," she admitted. "It wouldn't hurt to get my bloodwork checked."

That was an easy battle. Maybe she was feeling a little more cautious after dad's health problems earlier this year. She promised me she would call for an appointment right away. We chatted for a few minutes about work, the family and dad's health and then hung up. I felt better knowing she was going to get checked out, but I was still a little nervous about what could be wrong.

There were so many things that could be wrong. Stomach pain and fatigue were really broad complaints and it was easy to let my imagination run away with me. It could be something simple, like acid reflux, or it could be something serious like pancreatic cancer. See? I always jump to the worst possible conclusion.

I shook my head to clear my morbid thoughts and grabbed my bag. I was headed over to Shelby's apartment for the evening. My little sister and I were pretty close, even though we were very different. We both had our mom's nose and smile, but that was where the similarities ended. I had shoulder-length, caramel colored, straight hair and green eyes while Shelby got blond hair in ringlets all over her head and huge blue eyes with long, dark eyelashes. I was 5'6" with an average build and a gift for gaining a pound just by looking at cake. Shelby was 5'3" with a cute little figure and she could eat like a ranch hand and never gain an ounce. I was focused and practical and my dating life was non-existent; Shelby was flighty and free-spirited and always had a string of guys following her. It had been a long string of losers until last spring, when she met Wade. Now she was dating a great guy and I have to admit, I'm a little jealous.

I was headed over there to visit and let her practice her newly acquired massage therapy skills. She was finishing school and I was willing to be her practice dummy. It wasn't as easy when you were a nursing student- no one wanted to let you practice IVs on them. Shelby had dabbled in a number of careers before this latest venture. To pay the bills, she worked at a local diner called Joe's.

I got to Shelby's apartment and walked in without knocking. "Hello!" I called out as I came through the door.

Snickers came barreling out into the living room and rushed at me. Snickers was Shelby's incredibly spoiled pug, and she absolutely loved me, for no apparent reason. I didn't actually care for her, because she was snotty and slobbery and never obeyed. I got roped into dog-sitting her every so often, when Shelby managed to guilt me into it. It seemed the less I liked Snickers, the more she liked me, so I was about to get covered with dog hair and slobber.

Sure enough, she jumped up and pawed at me excitedly. I tried to pet her and push her back down to the floor at the same time. She was wagging her tail so hard her whole body was jerking around and she kept making snorting and snuffling noises that seem to go with having a flattened face. I thought she might go into a seizure, she was getting so worked up.

Shelby walked out of the kitchen with a plate full of spaghetti. "Hey, 'Lis," she said around a mouthful of noodles. "Want some?" she asked, gesturing at her plate with her fork. Snickers smelled food and immediately lost interest in me, running back over to Shelby to beg for food.

The spaghetti smelled delicious but with Shelby, you weren't always sure of the origin of the food. I figured I better find that out before I ate any of it.

"Did you make it?" I asked, not wanting to be rude, but not really knowing how else to ask.

She just laughed. "No, it was the special at work today and I brought home some of the leftover," she explained. I followed her into the kitchen where a restaurant carry out container sat on the counter still half full of noodles and sauce. “Tony is trying out Italian food.”

I grabbed a plate and scooped some pasta on to it. I popped it in the microwave to warm it up and grabbed a fork. I took a bite and practically groaned. I don’t know how, but Tony took a simple little dish like spaghetti and made it an absolute delicacy. This was miles better than anything I would have made at home.

“It’s good, huh?” Shelby said, with a grin. She worked at a diner in town so she had access to some pretty good food. Better her than me, she could eat delicious food and never gain weight. If I worked at Joe’s, I would weigh over 200 pounds.

“It’s amazing,” I replied, still shoveling food in my mouth. I think I was supposed to be eating slowly and savoring my food. Instead, I was devouring it like I was afraid someone was going to take it away from me.

“You should go out with Tony,” Shelby said. “He could cook stuff like this for you all the time.”

Tony was a cook at Joe’s and he was cute enough. He was tall and lanky and had an incredible smile. But I didn’t think it was appropriate to date a guy just for his culinary skills. Besides, after I got fat, he probably wouldn’t be interested anyway.

We finished our plates of pasta in silent appreciation of Tony’s amazing food. I dumped my plate and fork in the sink and grabbed a glass of water to wash it down.

"So, mom isn't feeling good," I said, trying to sound casual. No need to get everyone all riled up.

"What's wrong with her?" Shelby asked, with a raised eyebrow. She knew me well enough to know I was already worried.

"She's really tired a lot," I replied. "And her stomach is upset so she isn't eating much."

"What do you think it is?" Shelby asked me. I didn't need to scare her with my worst case scenarios, so I tried to downplay it.

"It could just be a stomach problem," I said calmly, using my professional nurse face and trying to sound unconcerned. "She said she would go to see Dr. Cullard and get it checked out."

"When did all this start?" she asked, looking a little upset. She must have thought she was being kept out of the loop.

"I just talked to them right before I came over here," I assured her. "Mom didn't even want to tell me, but dad told me she had been tired, so I kept bugging her."

"Well, tell me what they find out," she said, insistently. I agreed that I would tell her as soon as I heard anything.

We got down to the serious business of my massage and I was just starting to relax, when my phone chirped with a text message. I didn't really get too concerned, I got lots of text messages and they were usually just chatting. I would look at it later.

"Maybe it's from Jake," Shelby said, teasingly. My stomach fluttered at the mention of his name, even though I tried to convince myself to not react.

Shelby laughed out loud. "Do you know how tense you got as soon as I said 'Jake'?!" she chortled. "I guess Allie has a little crush."

"Shut up," I growled, because I didn't have any other rebuttal. And she was my little sister, so that was how a lot of our arguments ended.

Shelby went back to the task of un-knotting my neck and shoulders, still giggling softly to herself. I would throw a fit and stomp out, except I was minus some clothing at the moment. Besides, who wants to give up a free massage?

I got back to my house, relaxed and ready for bed. I remembered that I had heard a text message come in, so I pulled my phone out to look at it. My heart skipped a beat when I saw it was from Jake.

'*Had to take a pt in and you weren't there*' it said, with a sad face. I smiled, even though I tried not to.

'*I was getting a massage*' I texted back, with a smiley face. Getting a massage was a much better way to spend the evening than being at work. It was flattering to think that Jake was actually disappointed that he didn't get to see me when he brought a patient in. I never knew how seriously to take those statements, though.

'*From Shelby?*' he replied. It was late enough in the evening that a massage business wouldn't still be open.

'*Yep*' I texted back.

'*Good*' he replied. Once again, I wasn't sure what that meant. Was Jake actually jealous at the thought of me getting a back rub from another guy? Maybe I should fib and say it was a guy, to see how he reacted. Of course, I was terrible at lying, so I couldn't pull it off. Besides, I hated girls who played those kinds of games.

So I just replied with a pleasant '*Headed to bed. Have a good night shift*' and changed into pjs. I suddenly remembered I hadn't fed Oscar for a few days, so I walked back out into the living room. I turned the light on in the fish tank and Oscar came swimming excitedly up to the surface. He knew that meant it was feeding time. I threw in the pinch of flakes and he went to eating. I watched him furiously grabbing the little flakes and wondered if he ever worried that I was going to forget him entirely. I needed one of those automatic feeders like you got for hamsters. Except they don't make them for fish, so poor Oscar was dependent on his very forgetful owner. Maybe it was best I didn't have kids. I think you have to feed them more often than that.

Now that I had taken care of my fish, I could sleep peacefully. I brushed my teeth and gargled with a little extra mouthwash. The spaghetti was delicious, but it had a lot of garlic in it. No one was there to smell my breath when I woke up, but it still seemed like a good idea to fix the problem. What if I had a fire in the middle of the night and had to evacuate and didn't have time to grab a piece of gum? Then the fire department would be subjected to my garlic breath, and Jake was on duty tonight. Better safe than sorry.

My little house could get chilly at night, so I got my heating pad out and tucked it down in the foot of my bed. I liked to keep my toes nice and toasty when I slept. Shelby made fun of me, saying that sleeping with a heating pad meant I was an old lady. I didn't care. I snuggled down under the blankets, tucked my toes under the warm pad and drifted off to sleep.

The alarm rudely went off about ten minutes later. Or at least, that was how it felt. That massage made for a great sleeping pill. I smacked the alarm off and headed to the bathroom to get ready for work.

It was cold and cloudy, with a wind blowing leaves around in the gutter. I clutched my coat closed and scurried to the car. I started it and sat there, impatiently waiting for the heater to warm up. I wasn't acclimated to the cold yet. In January, I handled zero degree temps just fine but in October, the forty degree temps felt frigid.

I drove to work, and the heater finally got the car warmed up about the time I pulled into the hospital parking lot. I grabbed my bag and scurried into the building. This was a good day for staying curled up in a warm bed. But that wouldn't pay the bills.

I headed for my usual cup of coffee. I needed the caffeine and warmth both. With my hands wrapped around my coffee cup, I walked up to the nurses' desk, still feeling chilled.

"Hello, gorgeous," a low, delightful voice drawled. Jake was standing at the desk, looking handsome as always, and a shiver ran down my back that had nothing to do with the cold.

"Um, hi," I stammered in reply. "I didn't realize you guys were here." I could feel the heat rising in my cheeks, even though I was trying to act calm and collected.

A knowing grin spread across Jake's face and told me that he could see I was blushing. Which just resulted in me blushing even more.

"Thought we'd end the shift with one last drop-off to the ER," Jake laughed. He gestured into the room where Roger, the night shift nurse, was looking over a patient.

"And we wanted to see you, of course," Kent, Jake's partner, chimed in with a grin. I'm pretty sure he saw me blushing at the sight of Jake, too. Great. The guys at the station would have a field day with this. Jake was used to having women fall all over him, but I didn't really want to be part of the harem.

“What’s the patient?” I took the safe route of talking about work.

“Guy locked himself out of his house and tried to climb up to an open window,” Kent said. “Slipped off the window ledge and landed in the yard. He twisted his leg pretty bad and couldn’t get up, so he just yelled until someone heard him and called 911. Poor guy was out there for thirty minutes, and he’s freezing.”

At hearing that, I decided it was time to stop socializing and start working. I walked into the room to see what Roger needed for help.

“Hey Allie,” Roger said, looking up briefly. “Will you grab some blankets from the warmer?”

I had sort of figured that would be the first thing he needed, and I walked quickly back out to the blanket warmer and grabbed an armful of the warm blankets. They felt wonderful, and I wasn’t even hypothermic. I walked back in the room and started wrapping them around the guy laying on the gurney.

He looked up at me and attempted to smile. He was shivering from head to toe and his skin was pale. He had some blankets on him and I pulled them back to put the warm ones closest to his skin.

“Hi, I’m Allie,” I smiled at him as I was working on the blankets. He just nodded, grimacing when I got to the blankets on his legs. I gingerly worked the blankets loose to put the warm ones on. His left leg had an immobilizer on it and Roger was checking the circulation and sensation in his toes.

"This is Steve Rand," Roger said to me. "He's not having a very good morning."

"I hear you tried to turn into a popsicle," I joked. He half-smiled, but he still looked pretty miserable. Cold and in pain was not a fun combination.

Roger filled me in on the rest of Steve's information, including a temperature of only 95 degrees. We would give the warm blankets a few more minutes to work and then recheck it. We had a special warming blanket we could set up if his body temperature didn't come up quickly enough.

Jake and Kent came back in the room to say good-bye and good luck to Steve. Through chattering teeth, he thanked them for their help.

"Well, you've got the best nurse in town, now," Jake said, winking at me. "She'll have you fixed in no time."

I succeeded at not blushing this time, and smiled demurely at Jake. They waved to Roger and headed out the door. Just as they reached the door of the room, Jake turned back around and said, "I'm glad I got to see you, Allie." Then he was gone.

I was glad I had taking care of Steve to distract me from thinking about what Jake had said. Roger and I had finished up everything that needed to done for the initial assessment. I rechecked his temperature and it was now 96.1. An improvement at least. Now we needed to check out his leg a little closer.

Dr. Connelly walked in to the room as Roger was finishing report and getting ready to head home. Dr. Connelly was an Irishwoman to the bone, including her red hair and green eyes. She didn't have too bad of a temper, but she didn't put up with much. She only worked a few shifts a month at our ER. Her other job was at the state prison, so she always had good stories to tell. She was very no nonsense and could be a little blunt, but I got along with her okay.

"Colleen Connelly," she said to Steve, by way of introduction. I think she liked to skip saying the 'Doctor' part just to see if people would assume she was the nurse because she was female.

Steve didn't care if she was the cafeteria lady, he was in pain and needed some relief. After asking him about any drug allergies, she gave me an order to give him some morphine and a muscle relaxer. She also ordered an x-ray of the leg, but I wanted to get the pain meds in him before the x-ray tech started moving him around.

I drew up the morphine quickly and started injecting it slowly through his IV. I chatted with Steve as I pushed the drug, partly to be friendly and partly to slow myself down from giving it too fast.

Steve wasn't too chatty, mostly due to the pain, but he was friendly. He was pretty embarrassed about the morning's adventure. He hadn't called his work to tell them he wasn't coming in, because he didn't want to tell them what had happened. He lived alone, so no one was in his house to hear him yell. The neighbor lady had finally heard him, but she walked with a walker, so she couldn't do much except call 911.

I told Steve I could call his work for him and just say that he had fallen and was in the ER and that I couldn't give them any more information. Patient privacy laws, you know. He thought that sounded like a good cover story, and gave me the name and number of his manager.

The morphine was starting to kick in, and the x-ray tech was here to take Steve, so I stepped out to make the phone call and do some charting. I really didn't like charting, but I had learned to keep up on it as I went. It was easier to remember the events of the last twenty minutes that the entire last two hours. I jotted down the time I gave the medications and then went to the phone to call Steve's boss.

"Davis Lock and Key, how may I help you?" a friendly voice answered. I was thrown off for a moment. Steve worked for a locksmith? That would be ironic. Maybe I had dialed the number wrong.

"Could I speak to Jim Stanton, please?" I asked, just in case it was the right number. These days, everyone had caller ID, so when you were calling someone from a hospital phone, you didn't just hang up without saying anything. People got freaked out by that.

"Sure, one moment, please," she replied and then hold music came on. I tried to stifle a laugh. No wonder poor Steve didn't want to tell his work what had happened.

"This is Jim," a deep voice boomed through the phone.

"Hi, this is Allie in the ER at Brighton County," I introduced myself. "I'm sorry to have to call you, but Steve Rand is here with an injury and he wanted me to let you know that he won't be able to make it in to work today." I tried to keep my voice as bland as possible, to make it seem like the injury was no big deal.

"My goodness, what happened?" Jim asked with concern. Then, not waiting for a reply, he continued, "Is he okay?"

That gave me an easy out- I just answered the second question and skipped the first. "I can't give out much information, but he did say that I can tell you that he hurt his leg. We are doing an x-ray right now to see how badly it's hurt and he will be able to call you later with more information."

"Ok," Jim replied. He paused for a long moment, probably mulling over the situation. Then he said, "Thanks for calling. Tell Steve I hope he's okay."

"I will, sir. Thank you for your time," I finished and hung up the phone. That was nice that his boss was concerned about him and not just angry that he wasn't coming in to work. It was still going to be awkward when Steve had to tell them the details of his injury.

The x-ray tech had brought Steve back so I went to check on him. His temperature was now 97.1 and he said the morphine was helping his pain. I passed along the message from his boss and he looked relieved that there weren't more questions about what had happened.

"So," I said, pausing briefly to consider that maybe I should just keep my mouth shut, and then deciding against it, "you work for a locksmith?"

Steve looked downright sheepish. "I know," he groaned. "This is so embarrassing. I keep meaning to make an extra key and hide it outside, but then I forget. And I didn't want to admit it to anyone, so I wouldn't call to have someone from work come get me into my house." He ran his hands over his face in frustration.

I felt really bad for him. This was the kind of screw-up I could see myself making easily. It's so hard to admit when you're wrong, and then your foolish pride trips you up in a big way. My heart went out to the guy, but I didn't have any great words of wisdom for him. I just patted him on the shoulder and went out to the desk to see what Dr. Connelly had seen on the x-ray.

"Well, he broke it," she said, pointing at the image on the screen. "But it's a nice neat break as far as the bone is concerned. No need for surgery." That was a relief.

"He's going to be laid up for a while, though," she continued. "Those muscles are pretty shortened up from laying so long in that position. He's going to have a lot of pain and stiffness to work through."

That didn't sound like it was the least bit of fun. We had drugs to give for pain and for muscle spasm, but they could leave you pretty loopy. I guess sometimes you have to decide which of the two evils is lesser and pick it. When I had my wisdom teeth out, the pain pills they gave me definitely took away the pain, but they also left me basically comatose. I took them at night to sleep and otherwise I toughed it out with ibuprofen. I didn't have to worry about getting addicted to my painkillers, I couldn't stay awake long enough to abuse them.

Dr. Connelly went in to tell Steve about his leg and what his life was going to entail for the next week. He didn't look too thrilled with the news, but it could have been worse. I went back in the room to ask him if he had someone he could call to drive him home from the ER. He grimaced at that, and then thought for a minute.

"I don't really," he said. "I mean, everyone I know is at work and I don't want to ask someone to leave work just to come get me."

I didn't know if now was a good time to mention that we recommend people not be alone while they're on the drugs, just in case they have problems. Steve didn't sound like he had someone to sit at his house and watch over him, since he didn't even have a ride home.

Situations like this made me a little nervous for myself. If I was in the ER, who would I have to call? Shelby, obviously, and she would be happy to come get me and even stay with me. But what if Shelby was gone? What if she moved to Springfield to live with Wade? Who did I know and trust well enough to sit with me while I was zonked out on narcotics?

I shook my head, remembering that we weren't worried about me right now, we were worried about Steve. I tried to think of people who could help him.

"Do you have a pastor?" I asked. My pastor was always going around helping out people in the church, so it seemed it was part of the calling.

"Yeah," he said, sounding surprised. "I didn't even think of that. I can even stay with them, if I need to. They have an extra room in their house just for people like me."

I wasn't quite sure what he meant by that, and he must have seen the look on my face because he clarified, "Single people without someone to take care of them." Oh, those people.

"We have quite a few widows in our church," Steve explained. "When they were needing surgery or whatever, their kids live far away and they didn't have anyone to help them out at home. The pastor's son had gone away to college so they converted his room into a guest room for anyone that needed a place to stay for a few days. Then he and his wife can help them out if they need it."

Well that was a neat idea. Maybe I should mention it to my pastor and they could set up a room like that. It seemed like there were quite a few people who didn't live with anyone who could help take care of them.

That way, if Shelby married Wade, I had a backup.

Chapter 4

I woke up feeling extra ambitious, so I laced up my sneaks and went for a run. I cranked up the music loud enough to probably damage my hearing and pounded the pavement with fervor. Some days, my run was more like a shuffling jog, done with less enthusiasm and more feeling of paying penance for what I ate the night before.

I got back home, feeling extra healthy and a little virtuous, and hopped in the shower. I was drying off when I heard my phone ring. I grabbed it off the nightstand and saw it was mom calling.

"Hi mom," I said cheerfully. We spent so much time on the phone these days that I didn't get worried when she called anymore.

"Hi sweetie," she said, with a note of something not good in her voice. That made me instantly concerned.

"What's wrong?" I asked, bluntly. We weren't much for small talk and tiptoeing around things.

"Well, I went to Dr. Cullard yesterday," she started out. "He just called me this morning. I guess my blood levels are low and that's why I feel so tired."

"Mom, your blood levels of what?" I asked, trying not to lose my patience. There's about a thousand things to test a blood level for, so that statement didn't tell me much.

"Um, something with an 'H'," she said, uncertainly. "It carries oxygen, I guess."

"Oh, hemoglobin," I said, out of habit.

"Yes, that," she replied.

"Do you remember what it was?" I asked. It didn't really need to know the actual level, but it was hard to turn the nurse switch off.

"He didn't say," she replied. Well, the number didn't really matter but I was mildly curious. There was 'a little low' and then there was 'really low'. One just involved taking an iron supplement and one was a cause for concern.

"Why does he think it's low?" I asked. Mom was normally a healthy gal.

"He said I'm bleeding in my stomach," she said. "I guess that's what causing all my stomach problems."

"What kinds of problems were you having?" I asked. Now I was feeling guilty that I didn't ask her more questions when she had mentioned stomach problems.

"Well, my stomach hurts a lot," she said. "And I have to go to the bathroom quite a bit."

"Are you having loose stools?" I asked. It felt a little weird to play nurse with my own mother, but I knew my mom wouldn't volunteer up that kind of information.

“Um, sort of,” she said, hesitantly. “I don’t want to gross you out, but it smells really bad and looks funny.”

I wanted to laugh. After all the things that I had seen in the ER, I was not going to get grossed out by my mom discussing her bowel habits. I knew from my nursing experience that bleeding in the digestive tract led to very smelly, magenta-colored stools. There was a trademark smell to them, so the first time the patient went to the bathroom, you knew what was going on. Testing the stool for blood was just a formality.

“What does he think caused the bleeding?” I asked. A lot of things could bring on a GI bleed, and sometimes it’s tough to identify a cause.

“He said it’s from all the ibuprofen I’ve been taking,” she replied.

“Mom, why are you taking ibuprofen?” I asked. Mom didn’t have aches and pains that I knew of.

“My knee bothers me,” she replied, nonchalantly.

“How much do you take?” I asked. It usually takes a lot of ibuprofen before it causes stomach bleeding, although some people are more sensitive than others.

“Well, I take it every time it hurts,” she said, evasively.

“And how often is that?” I asked, patiently. I was used to patient interviews where I had to drag out every piece of information.

She hesitated for a long moment. "About every four hours," she finally said.

"Mom, you take ibuprofen every four hours?" I asked incredulously. That was a lot of ibuprofen. Now I was worried about her kidneys as well as her stomach.

"If I don't, it hurts me," she explained. She probably didn't realize how bad it was to take ibuprofen that much.

"Mom, why does your knee hurt so much?" I asked. I didn't remember her hurting it, although they didn't always tell me everything, because they didn't want me to worry.

"Oh, I'm just getting old," she said. "A few aches and pains are part of the territory."

"Mom, that much pain isn't normal with just aging," I explained. "Did you hurt it?"

"Well, I've had trouble with that knee for years," she replied. "It's just gotten worse over the last few months."

So she had started taking ibuprofen around the clock, which ate a hole in her stomach and caused bleeding that dropped her hemoglobin. Now that all made sense.

"Well, what did Dr. Cullard say to do?" I asked. This was the part where my nurse card came in. Dr. Cullard was a very nice doctor, but he had been in family practice in a small town for thirty years. I wasn't sure he was up to date on his medical knowledge, so I wanted to make sure he had come up with an appropriate plan of action.

"He wants me to start taking a couple pills for my stomach," she said. "One I take every morning and one I take with meals. And an iron tablet twice a day."

"What about the knee pain?" I asked. She needed to stop the ibuprofen, but she couldn't just be in constant pain.

"He wants me to go see another doctor," she said. "A surgeon. His name is Dr. Lytle. He said I need to see him right away, so I have an appointment tomorrow."

You had to love small towns. Everybody knew everybody, and Dr. Cullard probably had his secretary just call and make the appointment for mom right away. It was nice to have that kind of customer service. In bigger cities, a doctor would tell someone to go see a specialist and then wash their hands of it.

Dr. Cullard had told mom to switch to acetaminophen until she could see the surgeon, so that would help her stomach heal. She promised to call me when she heard what Dr. Lytle had to say and we got off the phone.

I called Shelby to fill her in. We had unofficially established a calling tree when dad had his heart attack that mom would call me and I would call the other kids. Shelby expected to be called first, and Andrew, our older brother, didn't mind being called second, as long as he got called.

Shelby didn't have much for questions. She usually trusted that I had covered all the important questions and let me handle it. I called Andrew next, and got voice mail. I wasn't leaving a message that contained all that info, so I just told him to call me. Then I called his wife, Nicole, figuring telling her was just as good. His wife was a sweetheart and my parents considered her another one of their children.

"Well, Allison Eloise, what a nice surprise," she answered, with an exaggerated Southern accent. She lived in Oregon, and had never even been to the South, but she liked to goof around.

"Hey, Nicole, how's it going?" I asked. She told me about the latest antics of their adorable twin girls, Cassie and Sammie. They had huge blue eyes, lots of blonde ringlets, and mischievous smiles. And they were usually getting into mischief.

I filled her in on mom and let her know I had left a message with Andrew. She told me he was out on a job site today, and probably couldn't hear his phone over the equipment. Andrew was a civil engineer, so he spent most of his days in an office. He was like a little kid again when he got to go out to the job site and see all the heavy equipment. It must be a boy thing.

After I got off the phone with Nicole, I was at a loss for what to do. I felt antsy now, and couldn't focus on anything. I didn't really have a reason to worry, but that never stopped me before. I was the queen of worrying.

I started in on laundry and housework, since it kept me busy and burned off some nervous energy. My mind kept wandering on me, even with the stereo cranked up to drown it out.

Finally, about eleven o'clock, I decided to go outside and burn some energy. Shelby was working the lunch shift at Joe's, so I figured I would go down there and get some lunch. The fridge was pretty bare anyways.

We were having a rare day of sunshine and slightly warmer weather, so I hopped on the bike. The season was about over, but I tried to drag it out as long as I could. I took the long way to Joe's, partly to burn off nervous energy and partly to offset the burger I was about to eat. I always went in there convinced I would get something healthy, but Joe's didn't have much for health food. They did have delicious fries, however.

I walked in and sat down at the bar. Shelby saw me and walked over with a glass of iced tea.

"Everything okay?" she asked, looking concerned.

"Yeah," I replied. "Just needed to get out of the house for a bit and I don't have much for food in my fridge."

She nodded understandingly. Shelby knew I was a worry wart. Everybody who knew me knew I was a worry wart. It was one of my greatest skills. A completely useless skill, but I kept at it anyway.

"Know what you want?" she asked. I didn't need to look at a menu, I knew it by heart.

"Cheeseburger and fries," I replied. She nodded and headed to the kitchen to turn in the order. I looked around the restaurant, which was busy as usual. A lot of business folks ate lunch at Joe's, because the food was good and the service was quick. I didn't see anyone I knew, which was unusual. I knew a lot of people in this town.

Tony came wandering out of the kitchen to say hi, like he usually did when I was there to eat. I complimented him on the spaghetti he had made the other day, and he grinned.

"Yeah, I make a mean pasta for being an Irishman," he joked. "Maybe there was some Italian blood way back in the line. Not that anybody would admit it if there was!"

I laughed at that. Italian blood or not, Tony definitely had Italian cooking down.

"Been out riding?" he asked me. Tony and I both enjoyed mountain biking, but on different levels. I liked trails and helmets and being able to see where I was going. Tony wore a helmet, mostly in case he suddenly slammed into a tree. He was a big fan of screaming downhill and jumping off of stuff. It was fun to watch but I was not interested in joining him. I got palpitations just watching him.

"I went up last week," I replied. "It's getting cold, though. Might be about time to put the bike up for winter." It was mid-October, which was actually late in the year for still having open trails, but the snow hadn't really hit yet so far.

"Be time to shred some powder soon," Tony said with a grin. This was a boring time of year for outdoor enthusiasts. It was too cold to do fun outside stuff, but there wasn't enough snow yet for the ski resorts to open. I always said I would use the downtime to catch up on the stuff on my 'To Do' list, like learning Spanish and organizing the storage in my basement. Yet, I never did.

Shelby walked back up with my burger and set the plate in front of me. There was a plastic cup with some kind of sauce in it sitting next to the fries.

"Try that stuff," Tony said, gesturing to the cup. "It's a new fry sauce I'm trying out."

I looked at the cup of thick, pink-colored and creamy sauce. I was a little nervous to try it, even though Tony made great stuff. I was usually just a ketchup girl when it came to fries. But Tony and Shelby were looking at me expectantly, so I picked up a fry, dipped it in the sauce and took a bite. It was amazing.

"That's really good!" I gushed. "What's in it?"

Tony laughed. "Secret recipe," he replied. "So you like it?"

I had already shoveled in three more fries dipped in the sauce. I nodded enthusiastically while I chewed.

"Good," he said. "Glad to know you approve." He flashed his incredible smile at me as I continued to devour my fries. Tony had seen me eat before, so I didn't have to act shy. Besides, since he was the cook, he liked to see people enjoying his food.

"Well, whatever the secret is, I'd say you have a winner on your hands," I told him. I didn't want to know what was in it because it was super creamy, which I'm sure did not translate to low calorie. Some things it was just better not to know.

Someone in the back yelled for Tony, so he sauntered back toward the kitchen, tossing a 'see ya' over his shoulder. I had polished off my fries so I started working on my cheeseburger.

I ate my burger a little slower than I had eaten my fries, at least. Shelby hung out and chatted with me for a bit. We talked about what might be wrong with mom's knee, even though at this point, everything was just speculation.

"Doing anything fun this weekend?" I asked her. She had more of a social life than I did, usually.

"Wade is coming down to visit," she said with a smile. Shelby had met Wade when he was the nurse taking care of our dad earlier this year. They had been dating since then, and he was a huge step up from the guys she used to date. I was happy to see it was still going strong. He lived 100 miles away, which can be hard on a dating life.

I said good-bye to Shelby and headed out the door. I felt better now, although, I wasn't sure why. Maybe Tony's secret recipe included Xanax. I rode home and stashed the bike in the garage. My little house had a small, detached garage out back. I used it for storage, since extra space was at a premium in the house. I still had some summer stuff that I needed to box up and get out to the garage. More of those things I was always intending to do. Well, today was the perfect day. It had been sunny and brisk, but now it was clouding up and getting cold. Maybe we were getting ready for some snow.

I went through the house collecting the scattered summer gear- flip flops, camping chairs, backpack, five different pairs of sunglasses. Summer was my favorite season and it made me sad to pack all that stuff away. It had been a short summer, or at least it felt like it. I had made several trips to visit my parents, which meant I spent less days playing in the sun. I looked at all the bottles of sunscreen and wondered if they were still good if I stored them for a year. I decided to take a chance and tossed them into the box as well. If I didn't die of skin cancer, I could die of cancer from expired sunscreen, right?

I was carrying the boxes out to the garage when I overheard the neighbors arguing. Jim and Cathy were a very nice couple in their fifties, but they loved to fight. At least that was how it seemed, as much as they did it.

"You can't put it there, it looks stupid," Cathy snapped at Jim. They were hanging their Halloween decorations, apparently.

"It doesn't matter," Jim growled back. "It's only going to be there for a couple weeks. Why are we even bothering with this?"

"Well, I wanted to do it earlier!" Cathy shrieked. "You're the mule headed lunk that refused to put them up!"

"I hate Halloween. Dumbest holiday ever. Bunch of greedy kids in stupid costumes," Jim muttered.

Cathy ignored him and directed him to hang the witch decoration in the tree. She didn't seem to care that Jim didn't like Halloween, he was getting in on the fun anyway.

"Jeez, now every time I see this, I'll think your mother is here to visit," Jim cracked as he hung the witch. I tried not to giggle at that. They hadn't noticed me yet, and I wanted to stay out of the argument.

"Keep it up and I'll invite her to stay for a month," Cathy threatened as I headed back to the house. Jim pantomimed hitting his head with the hammer he was holding. I made it back inside without being spotted. They were always very friendly to me, but when they were fighting, it was just awkward for me to be in the middle of it.

Marriage was a funny thing, sometimes. It seemed like married people fought with each other more than they fought with anyone else. Maybe that was part of the marriage deal. You agreed to be each other's punching bag, so you could get all your frustrations out and didn't end up fighting with everyone else. Yet another thing about marriage I did not understand.

I decided the colder weather was a good excuse for making chili, and since my kitchen was looking like Mother Hubbard's cupboard, I needed to make a grocery trip. I grabbed a jacket and hopped in the car.

The store wasn't too busy, which was a good thing. I could get pretty distracted when I was shopping and I had problems with not looking where I was going. If the store was crowded, that was just more people for me to run into with my cart. I got all the stuff for chili, as well as the usual milk/bread/fruit basics. I rationalized that a cornbread mix was a necessary component for making chili, and, of course, I needed butter and honey to put on the cornbread.

I got to the checkout with a full cart, and started unloading it on to the counter. The lady in line ahead of me was using about a dozen coupons, so it was taking a while. I leafed through a magazine while I waited, trying not to be impatient. I skimmed a health and fitness magazine, seeing if they had any information I couldn't live without. I subscribed to a magazine like this, and it seemed like their articles were the same thing, rewritten slightly, each month. All of the pictures were of perfectly toned, tanned twenty-year-olds in workout gear that was practically underwear. I decided I didn't need them making me feel worse about my body, so I stuck the magazine back in the rack.

I got through the checkout and lugged my bags to the car. I drove home as scattered little drops of rain hit my windshield. The weather was definitely turning toward winter. I parked the car and loaded all of my bags of groceries in both hands. It really would have made more sense to make two trips, since I had so many bags. However, I didn't always do things the way that made sense. I walked quickly toward the door, hands cramping, feeling the bags sliding as I hurried. I pushed open the door lever with my elbow and stepped into the kitchen, with my hands going numb. I dumped all the bags on the floor and stood there for a minute, rubbing my fingers as the circulation returned.

I put away the food and took out the crock pot. I liked to simmer my chili for a good twelve hours, so if I started it now, I could eat it tomorrow. I started dumping in ingredients, stirred it all together and set the crock pot on low.

I had bought a can of chicken rice soup for supper tonight. Those overly pious nutrition experts would say there was too much sodium in canned soup, but cooking an entire meal for one person was just too much work sometimes. I dumped the soup into a bowl and stuck it in the microwave to heat it up.

I wandered into the living room and turned on the TV. I needed a little mindless entertainment to go with my dinner. This was good weather for curling up on the couch and spending the evening doing nothing. I heard the microwave ding and went back to get my supper. I settled in on the couch and savored my warm soup. Soup just always tasted better when it was cold outside. I finished my meal and snuggled up in a fleece blanket to watch the rest of the TV show.

I woke up just after midnight to an infomercial on TV. I shook my head groggily and clicked the TV off. I shuffled to my bedroom, tumbled into bed and promptly fell asleep again.

I woke up the next morning bright and early. That would be the advantage of falling asleep by 9 o'clock at night, I guess. I laid snuggled under the covers for a few minutes, savoring the luxury of not having to set an alarm or get out of bed right away. I loved my job, but days off were still a wonderful thing.

I finally crawled out of bed and headed to the kitchen to make a pot of coffee. It was chilly in my little house this morning. I wrapped my thick robe around me tighter and went to turn up the thermostat. The chili was bubbling in the crock pot and the house smelled delicious. I briefly considered having chili for breakfast, since it was a hot meal and already cooked, but decided to hold off until lunch. I had my usual toast and some yogurt.

Mom's appointment with the surgeon wasn't until 10 o'clock, so I had over two hours to kill. I turned on the laptop to check email and pay an online bill. Of course, then I wandered on to Facebook and spent close to an hour looking at the silly stuff people post. It was a good way to kill time and entertain myself so I didn't just sit and worry. Videos of howling puppies and teenagers falling off of stuff were just the distraction I needed.

My phone ringing startled me. I looked at the screen and didn't recognize the number, but it was the same prefix as my parents' number, so I decided I better answer it.

"Allison, it's mom," I heard my mom say, but it sounded weird, like she was far away.

"And I'm Dr. Lytle," a male voice chimed in. "We have you on speaker phone here at my office. Can you hear okay?"

My heart started racing and my mind was racing even faster, wondering what could possibly be so wrong that the doctor himself would call me while my mom was still in his office? Luckily, Dr. Lytle jumped right to the point.

"Allison, your parents tell me you're a nurse and they want you to be involved with decisions," he said."I figured the easiest way was to just have the conversation with you on the line. Then we don't have to repeat anything."

I was still nervous about what was so serious that I needed to make medical decisions, but I just replied, "Um, that sounds good."

"Your mom's knee has old scar tissue in it, that's built up over the years," he explained. "We need to go in and clean it out, and she'll have a lot less pain. None, hopefully, after it heals up."

So far this sounded exactly like what I had thought he would say, but I was still on edge.

"The procedure is an arthroscopy, so it doesn't require us to open up her knee. While it's not a major surgery, it still requires a little bit of specialty. We used to send people out to another, larger hospital to have this done. But we've started trying something new."

He paused, and I figured this was the part my parents wanted me involved in. Dr. Lytle continued, "There is an orthopedic surgeon, Dr. Steitler, in Marbleton who does hundreds of these procedures. Once a month or so, he comes here to Madison and works with me and the OR crew here, doing these less invasive procedures. The benefit is that she doesn't have to travel, she gets to have the hometown hospital staff she already knows, and it costs less."

I thought that sounded good, but I knew he also had to discuss the downside. There were always pros and cons, and medical ethics required him to disclose all of both before mom made a decision.

"Now, if there are complications, of course, we're in Madison, and we can't handle as much here," he went on to explain. "I make rounds on Betty after surgery and do her follow up visits. If I have any concerns or questions, I can call Dr. Steitler anytime. If something major happened, like an infection or bleeding, that we couldn't treat here, we would have to transport her to a larger hospital."

I knew these types of orthopedic procedures were very common and rarely had complications. I also knew that the hospital in Madison was excellent, even though it wasn't very big, and I trusted the staff there. Marbleton was 80 miles north of Madison, and it would be a lot easier for everyone if mom could stay in Madison for all of this. But, it wasn't really my decision to make. I wished I could see my mom, so I could read her expression.

"So, we're discussing this as an option for having the surgery here," Dr. Lytle said. "Do you have any questions?"

I couldn't think of anything right off the top of my head. It sounded like a pretty good deal, at least so far.

"Mom, what do you think?" I asked. I didn't want to talk her into something she didn't really want to do.

"I want to do it here," she said, emphatically. Well, that answered that question. Mom had made up her mind.

"Ok," I replied. "But don't worry about it being a problem if you go to Marbleton," I started to assure her.

She cut me off. "I appreciate it, Allison, but I really want to stay here. Springfield hospital was great with your dad, but I hated being so far away from home. I don't want to be in the hospital at all, but if I have to stay a few days, I would rather do it here."

"Dr. Steitler is well-renowned for this procedure," Dr. Lytle interjected. "You can look him up on the hospital website. He's excellent at what he does."

It sounded like we had reached a decision. I figured I better ask dad, just to make sure we were all on board with this.

"Dad, what do you think?" I asked.

"No point in going clear up there when we have everything we need right here," dad replied. That was about what I thought he would say, and I completely agree with him.

"Well, I guess we have our decision," I said to Dr. Lytle. "Now, when will Dr. Steitler be down next?"

"He actually has an OR day next Monday," Dr. Lytle replied. "His schedule was filled, but his first case of the day just had to cancel. So, she can go next Monday morning at 7 a.m. Her hemoglobin is still low, but the surgery has minimal blood loss, so we can still go ahead."

It was Friday morning, and my head swam a bit, realizing my mom would have surgery in three days.

"Wow, that's quick," I said, a little dazed. I was frantically trying to figure out a schedule and when I would be able to get to Madison to see my mom. I knew she didn't really need me there, and I didn't want to treat her like she wasn't capable of going through a surgery without me.

"Allison?" mom's voice broke into my thoughts. "I hate to be a bother, but I would really like it if you could be here. Do you have to work?"

I was startled to hear my mom ask me to be there. They were usually trying to tell me I didn't have to come. Of course, I never listened to them.

"No," I replied. I did have to work on Tuesday, but I was going to leave that part out for now. I would find someone to cover my shift. My mom had asked me to come be with her while she had surgery, and so I was going to be there. Besides, we got emergency medical leave for immediate family members.

"I'll call you later and we can make plans," I said. Dr. Lytle didn't want to hear all of the planning, and he probably had another patient to see. "Is there anything else to discuss, Dr. Lytle?" I asked.

"No, if we're all in agreement, I'll call the hospital and have them put her on the schedule for Monday morning," he replied. "I'll give her a folder with information on what to do before surgery and what to expect afterwards. I'll give her my home phone number so if she has any questions over the weekend, she can call and ask me."

I had to smile at that. Not many doctors would give a patient their home number to call over the weekend. Small town doctors still worked in a different era, but it was nice for me. I was sure that I would think of all kinds of questions to ask later.

I thanked the doctor and hung up the phone. Now I had to wait until mom got done with the doctor before I could call her and plan the next week. I logged on to my hospital's website to check the schedule. I needed to find someone to cover a shift for me, and I could take care of that while I was waiting.

Besides, it was best to keep my mind occupied, so it didn't run away on me.

Chapter Five

I talked to Jesse and he agreed to work for me on Tuesday, but he wanted me to work this Saturday for him as a trade. I figured that was fair enough and it wasn't like I had any exciting plans anyway. With the colder weather, I tended to stay at home more, at least until there was snow on the ground. I was just glad to get my shift covered so I could be with my mom for surgery.

I dished up a steaming bowl of chili for lunch, and then remembered I was going to bake cornbread to go with it. Oh well, I had a whole pot of chili here, I could make the cornbread this afternoon and have it with my supper bowl of chili. I stirred in some cheese and crumbled some tortilla chips on the top and dug in.

I had called Shelby and Andrew, but got voice mail on both of them. I left a brief message that mom was having surgery in Madison on Monday, and I was pretty sure both of them would be calling me for more information once they got the message. I decided to spend the afternoon reorganizing my closet, so my cold weather clothes were easier to get to. It was also a good opportunity to decide which clothes I hadn't worn in over a year and needed to take to the Salvation Army.

With my closet all straightened around and my pan of cornbread cooling on the counter, I was feeling pretty accomplished. My phone rang and it was Shelby, as expected, wanting to know more about mom's surgery.

I filled her in on Dr. Steitler and that mom could have surgery at home and she thought it was a great idea as well.

"So, she actually asked you to be there, huh?" Shelby inquired. We were both used to our parents insisting they didn't need help.

"Yeah, and I got my shift covered so it's all good," I replied. "I'm glad I can go. It will make me less antsy."

"I'm glad you're going, too," Shelby said. "You can keep me posted. Dad probably wouldn't call anyone until she was already back home."

I laughed, but it was sort of true. He was always saying 'I didn't want to worry you' to me, which just resulted in me worrying more.

I heard Snickers going nuts all of the sudden, and then Shelby said, "Wade's here, I better go." We hung up and I suddenly felt a little lonely. It was supposed to be date night and I was sitting at home alone with nothing but a TV and cornbread for company.

Well, I was willing to make the most of the situation, so I changed into comfy sweats, cut a huge piece of still warm cornbread, smothered it in butter and honey and then settled on the couch to enjoy my carb-fest and watch TV.

I woke up rested and refreshed with the alarm the next morning, mostly because I went to bed at 9 o'clock. Just as well, a twelve hour shift went better if I had lots of sleep the night before.

The car windshield was frosted over, but I really hated scraping the windows, so I cranked up the defroster and waited for it to melt the frost off. My garage, sadly, was too small to hold my car. I'm not sure what they put in it when they built it, because I don't think cars were ever that small. Maybe it held a buggy instead. My house was old enough, that was a possibility.

The windshield finally had a hole cleared and I figured I could see to safely drive, so I headed off to the hospital. I got to work and filled my cup of coffee, as always. I walked up to the desk to see the EMT's transferring a patient to the gurney in the trauma room, so I headed in there right away. The general mood in the room was pretty relaxed, so I could tell the injuries weren't serious.

"Allie, this is Jason Davis," Sandy, the night shift nurse, said to me. The guy looked over toward me, at least as much as he could with the C-collar on, and smiled.

"Jason was driving to work today, and he ran in to a tree," Greg, one of the EMTs said with a wicked grin. Jason grimaced at the mention of that, and tried to shake his head in disbelief.

"That was the dumbest thing I've ever done," he sighed. "I can't believe it."

I didn't ask, just waited for someone to fill me in on what Jason had done that was so dumb. I was pretty sure it wouldn't be anything too shocking for an ER nurse, in fact, it might be something I'd heard before.

"Jason doesn't like to scrape the windshield," Greg continued. "So he just let the defrost run until a hole was cleared off and then he tried to drive. He was turning a corner and cut it too close, since he couldn't really see out the right side of the car. Car jumped the curb and smashed in to a tree.

Jason just groaned as Greg told the story. I didn't see any obvious injuries and no one seemed that worked up over the accident. I sort of wondered why he came to the ER after a minor fender bender.

Greg didn't let me wonder for long. "The lady who owns the tree called 911. When we got there, Jason was still in the vehicle and looked a little dazed. He couldn't remember if he hit his head or if he lost consciousness at all, but when we questioned him, he didn't know what day it was. Just to be on the safe side, we brought him in."

Well, that made a little more sense. Maybe Jason had hit his head, and he might have a head injury or a neck injury. Better safe than sorry.

"Of course," Greg continued, "after we were on our way in, he informs me that he never knows what day it is unless he's looking at a calendar."

"Or it's Sunday, and I'm watching football," Jason interjected.

I laughed at that. I had trouble with what day it was myself, sometimes. We always referred to our last shift in a stretch as 'my Friday', which got me messed up about when the actual Friday was.

Well, Jason was here now and we were going to check him out thoroughly, just in case. He looked a little uncomfortable with the C-collar and backboard on, but we had to have his spine cleared by the doctor before we could take them off.

Sandy finished up the details on report and then headed home. Greg and Josh finished their EMS report and stopped to say good-bye to Jason before they headed back to the station for shift change.

"Good luck, man," Greg said, grinning. Then he winked at me and said, "Your boyfriend is working today. Maybe you'll get to see him later."

I willed myself not to blush, successfully this time, and just said, "Have a good day off, guys." They waved and headed out the door. I turned my attention to Jason, asking him the usual questions about pain, numbness or tingling. Then I moved on to the health history questions, which didn't take long either. He was a fairly healthy young man, had asthma as a child and his appendix out when he was twelve.

Dr. Wallace walked in the room as I was finishing up. He seemed to be in a pleasant mood this morning. Usually, he didn't go in a patient's room until I specifically went out to the desk to hand him a chart and tell him the patient was ready. He introduced himself to Jason and asked him what had happened.

Patients can get frustrated with us when three different people ask them the same questions. But a lot of times, they remember something more each time. And sometimes, if they aren't being honest to start with, we get a different story each time. It just helps us get a more complete picture of the patient, even if it is a little annoying.

Jason just really didn't want to have to admit what he had done another time, but he complied. He sort of skimmed past the part where he couldn't see out of his windshield very well, but Dr. Wallace didn't let him get away with it.

"Were you peephole driving?" he asked bluntly. Jason looked bewildered at that expression.

"What's that?" he asked.

"When you only have a peephole to see through, because you didn't scrape off the whole windshield," Dr. Wallace replied.

Jason looked sheepish, and admitted, "I guess. But I had a pretty good hole, it was about this big!"

He held his hands up to demonstrate the size of the area he could see through and my stomach sank a little. That was about the size of the 'peephole' I had when I left for work today. I guess I better start scraping my windshield. I didn't want to be in here explaining to my co-workers why I hit a tree with my car.

Dr. Wallace got down to business, checking over Jason's neck and back so we could take him off the backboard. Jason was slim enough that I could turn him easily. With the more rotund ones, I was turning them toward me and wondering if they were going to come off the edge of the cart and land on the floor, with me squished underneath.

Dr. Wallace went through a check of his pupils and reflexes and it looked like Jason was going to be okay. The police officers had shown up to ask him about his little accident this morning, so we let them go in and chat with him while we finished up his discharge paperwork.

"Triage," I heard Tracy call out. Linda was already headed for the window, so I just kept charting and finished my coffee. Looked like it might be a busy one today.

By 10 o'clock, we had acquired a sore throat, an abdominal pain, a sprained ankle and a dementia patient that fell at the nursing home. Scott came walking in to work and stopped to look over the patient board for a minute.

"Anything exciting?" he asked me. Scott was a paramedic on the fire department for twenty years before he came to the hospital, so none of the minor medical cases we had today were going to be 'exciting' for him.

"No, but the day is young," I joked. He laughed and went to put his bag in the break room.

"I need some hands in here!" I heard Linda cry out from room 8. I rushed into the room to see Linda standing on the patient's left side, holding down his left arm, and reaching across to hold down his right hand. This put her within biting distance for the patient, and he was trying to take a chunk out of her arm.

I grabbed the patient's right arm for her, so she could move out of harm's way. This was our dementia patient, and he didn't understand what was going on, but he wasn't going down without a fight. His IV was in his right hand, and he had been trying to pull it out. He was downright scrawny, with paper thin skin and fragile little veins, so we wanted to keep the IV safe.

For such a frail little thing, he sure was strong. I felt his bony fingers closing down on my wrist and instinctively pulled my hand loose, just in time. He had hit his knee when he fell, so one leg was hurting him and he wouldn't move it. The other leg was swinging and kicking at anyone who got close enough.

Any attempts to calm the patient down were futile. He had decided we were enemy soldiers, 'probably Japs', trying to hold him prisoner and he was going to fight to the death. I was starting to worry that Linda and I were going to lose this battle, when Scott walked through the door.

Scott is over six feet tall, with a shaved head and white goatee. He has broad shoulders, burly arms, and a couple tattoos. He looks a little out of place in the ER, but today, that was a good thing.

The patient saw Scott and stopped moving. He stared at him in awe for a moment, then cried out, "Thank you, sweet Jesus, the cavalry is here!" Scott smirked at us and walked over to the patient's bedside.

"How do you do, sir?" he asked in a solemn voice.

"Get these Japs off me before they tie me to a post and shoot me!" the patient yelled out. Since he had stopped squirming, Linda and I gingerly let go of his arms and stepped back from the gurney. Scott stepped up and reached down to shake the patient's hand.

"Thank you," the patient gushed to Scott. "You saved my life!"

"Happy to help, sir," Scott maintained his solemn face through the whole ordeal. Linda and I were too stunned to say anything.

"How about if I take care of this gentleman today?" Scott said to Linda, making it sound like a casual suggestion.

Linda didn't have any ego issues about letting the paramedic take over, and she eagerly handed him the chart. She rattled off the details of his injury and health history, and then, just to be a smart aleck, she saluted Scott before she left the room. I stifled a giggle and followed her.

"Is everything ok in there?" Dr. Wallace asked, pretending to look concerned. I wasn't buying it, he hadn't bothered to come in when Linda was calling for help.

"Scott has saved the day," Linda replied. We both laughed at that, and Dr. Wallace looked a little confused. We just let him wonder and moved on to the next patient.

Some of our nurses didn't like having a paramedic working in the ER. I don't know why, Scott was fantastic at what he did. I guess it was an ego thing, since nurses went to more schooling than paramedics, they thought they automatically knew more. But most of what I learned didn't come from school, it came from actually working. As far as I was concerned, Scott had a 20-year degree.

I took the discharge papers in to the sore throat patient. Dr. Wallace had written a prescription for an antibiotic, and told her to use ibuprofen and saline gargles for the pain. She didn't seem too happy with that, and I got to be in the middle of things.

"I am in a lot of pain!" she wailed. "I need something stronger for pain."

She hadn't yet said what it was she wanted, but I'm sure if we asked her, she would be able to request the drug by name. She came to the ER about once a month with some type of pain or another.

"Ibuprofen is strong enough for a sore throat," I told her, trying not to get drawn into the argument.

"Well, I also have a really bad headache," she added quickly, "and a stiff neck. And ibuprofen isn't going to be strong enough."

"Dr. Wallace ordered ibuprofen," I told her firmly. "That's all you're going to get."

She flopped back on the gurney and started crying. "No one understands how much pain I have!" she wailed, theatrically. "No one wants to help me."

She sat up abruptly and said, "Why don't you want to help me?" in a plaintive voice.

"Kerry, you're on the red flag list," I reminded her. The red flag list was how we kept track of drug seekers, and once a person came in looking for pain pills often enough, they ended up on the list. They knew a lot of tricks- they would come on varying shifts to get different doctors, they had different complaints each time, they even drove to other towns to try to get drugs in those ERs.

Kerry knew she was on the list, but she still tried every so often. She struck out today because the doctor and both of the nurses knew her well. I wished she would find a better use for all that perseverance. If she had that much tenacity for something productive, there would be no stopping her. Sadly, she seemed to lack any direction in her life, and the only driving ambition she had was driven by addiction.

Kerry finally admitted defeat and slumped out the door, still pouting. Two other young people, sitting in the waiting room, jumped up and looked at her expectantly when she walked out. She just shook her head and they both deflated a little. It looked like Kerry was trying to score something for more than just herself. I wondered if we would see one of the other two later tonight, after the shift change.

It was almost two o'clock and we were finally starting to clear out the rooms, when the EMS radio went off.

"Structure fire, three occupants. All units respond." The words hung hauntingly in the air. We all looked at each other, apprehension in our eyes. It could possibly be a small fire and everyone would be fine, but somehow, we knew that wasn't the case. Just a gut feeling.

The radio continued with more details. It was an older mobile home in a park on the edge of town. The neighbor calling it in was certain that the couple and their son were all in the trailer, because their vehicle was in the driveway. She was especially concerned about the son, who was twelve years old and had Down's syndrome.

After a few minutes, we heard the fire engine respond that they were on scene, followed by a second engine and the ambulance. Then the radio was silent, and the next thing we would hear would be the ambulance calling report. It would be a while for that, though.

We continued on with finishing up the patients that we had, but we all had an uneasy air around us. I said a silent prayer for the safety of everyone involved. Trailer fires were scary, because they burned up so quickly. I tried to keep busy and not think about it too much.

After what seemed like an eternity, the radio came to life with the ambulance crew calling. I walked over to the radio and said, “This is ER, go ahead.”

“We’re coming in with all three occupants,” a serious voice came over the radio. I recognized it as Jake’s, but it was not his usual friendly tone. “The boy is unharmed, but very anxious. Both parents are unconscious, probable smoke inhalation.”

I could hear a child screaming out in the background. It had to be the son, and he probably didn’t understand what was going on. Jake continued with the major details on each adult- both had a heartbeat but were requiring assistance to breathe. They had been found in their bedroom, near the largest part of the blaze, and had singe marks on their faces and hands.

Just as I thought Jake was finishing report, he added on, “And Kent needs to be seen as well. There was an additional explosion as we were leaving the structure and he got struck with a piece of metal.” He gave an ETA of five minutes and then the radio was silent.

Dr. Wallace looked grim. This was three serious patients at one time, plus a distraught child. I wasn’t feeling too confident in how well this would go. But Dr. Wallace surprised me again.

“I’m calling Springfield right away,” he said, decisively. “This is more than we can handle and we are going to have to ship these patients.”

I was relieved to hear him say that, because this really was more than we could handle. Our little hospital didn't have pulmonologists or intensivists, and it sounded like these two were going to need both. Dr. Wallace was already on the phone with the intensivist in Springfield, giving him a heads up on the patients.

I had opened up the trauma room as well as the cardiac room next to it. They were our largest rooms, and had the resuscitation equipment in them. I hoped we wouldn't have to use it, but I wanted it handy if we did.

The ambulance pulled in and two guys in bunkers jumped out of the back. They brought out one gurney, with a man on it, and started wheeling it toward the door. As the automatic door slid open, they pushed the gurney toward me and Scott and said, "Here, take this." Then they turned back to the ambulance to get the second one.

Scott and I grabbed the gurney and wheeled it into the first room. Linda stayed at the door and waited for the second one to come in. We were getting the monitor connected to our patient when I heard the second cart go by the door. The boy was walking along behind it, wailing, "Mama! Mama! Mama!" It was absolutely heart wrenching to hear the terror in his voice. He couldn't understand exactly what was going on, but he knew enough to know something was seriously wrong.

We had our patient on high flow oxygen and Scott was using the ambu –bag to assist him with breathing. He had an IV and fluids going, so I grabbed some lab tubes and a needle. We had to check some blood levels to determine how serious their condition was. The room smelled like smoke and burned hair. It was a good thing I had a strong stomach. I got the blood I needed and walked out to the desk to get it labeled and sent to lab right away.

Kent was sitting in a chair in the hallway, holding his left arm and groaning. Jake was crouched beside him, with a concerned look on his face. I walked over to see what Kent's injuries were.

"Hey, Kent, what happened?" I asked.

"The propane tank on the BBQ grill blew up," he groaned, painfully. "A piece of something metal slammed into my arm."

He still had his bunker jacket on, as well as a shirt underneath it. I wasn't sure why he sat in the hallway, maybe he was afraid what we would do to him if he went in a room.

"Kent, we need to get you in a room and get your jacket off," I said gently. He grimaced at the mention of that, but nodded grimly and gingerly got to his feet. Jake was at his side, helping him stand, and looking almost nervous. He walked into the closest room with Kent and helped him sit on the edge of the gurney. Then he carefully removed his bunker jacket, trying to move the arm as little as possible.

His t-shirt was still covering part of the arm, but the part I could see had a pretty impressive bruise forming already. I grabbed a pair of trauma shears and cut away the sleeve of the shirt. The bruise ran the length of his upper arm, from the shoulder almost to the elbow.

"Does anything else hurt?" I asked him as I looked him over. When one injury was really painful, it could distract from other injuries, even though they might be more serious. I didn't see anything major, some minor scrapes on his hands and the side of his face. Kent shook his head, still grimacing.

"No, but that arm hurts enough," he muttered. I asked him to wiggle his fingers and he was able to do that, as well as feel me touching him. He was looking a little pale, so we helped him lay back on the gurney and elevated the arm on a pillow.

"I'll go get you an ice pack," I said, turning to leave the room.

"I'll do it," Jake said quickly. "You need to go back to the guy."

I had almost forgotten about the man in the first room, I was so focused on Kent. Kent's injury was much less serious, but I knew him, and somehow that made it more important in my mind. I was glad Jake brought me back to reality.

"Thanks," I said, as I headed back toward my patient. Scott was still in the room with him, so I knew he was in good hands. Dr. Wallace was in there, doing a cursory assessment, so he could call back to Springfield for Life Flight.

"No change," Scott said to me. "Might want to step next door and see if Linda needs you." He gave me a pointed look that told me Linda had her hands full with a patient and the distraught son. I nodded and walked into the next room.

Linda was standing next to the patient, holding an oxygen mask over her face. The boy was sobbing and trying to climb on the gurney with his mom. He kept pulling on her arms, and Linda was trying desperately to keep him from pulling the IV out. She looked up at me in desperation.

"His name is Timmy," she said, and that was all I needed for now.

"Timmy," I said, reaching out for his hand. "Timmy, it's okay. We're going to help her." I kept grabbing and holding his hand each time he tried to pull on his mom, and kept repeating, "Timmy, it's okay," over and over.

Of course, I didn't know for sure that it was okay, but right now Timmy just needed to be consoled. I repeated the phrase at least a dozen times, in an almost sing-song voice, and finally Timmy began to calm down. His heaving sobs began to subside but he still looked scared.

"Timmy, if I get a chair, do you want to sit right next to mom?" I asked.

He nodded vigorously. I placed his hands over her hand that didn't have an IV and instructed him to stay right there and hold her hand while I got the chair. He grabbed her hand and squeezed it tight. I got a chair from the corner of the room and brought it up behind him.

“Timmy, sit right here and hold mom’s hand while we help her get better, ok?” I told him. He nodded, still looking wide-eyed, and sat in the chair.

‘Thank you’ Linda mouthed to me over the top of the patient. She was drawing blood as well, just like I had. She filled the tubes and walked out to the desk to send them to lab. I stayed in the room with Timmy, just in case he got agitated again. He looked so frightened, it just broke my heart.

Linda came back in and motioned that she was okay and I could go now. I quickly peeked in to room 1 and Scott still had everything under control. I hurried back down to Kent’s room, where he was still groaning and Jake was still looking worried.

“Did Dr. Wallace come in yet?” I asked. He was currently at the desk on the phone with the hospital in Springfield, and I wasn’t sure he remembered that Kent needed to be seen.

“No,” Jake answered. “But I know the other guys are more serious.”

That was true, but we didn’t need to leave Kent in misery. I could help the doctor out and move things along a little quicker.

"Kent, are you allergic to anything?" I asked. Important to know that before we gave him any drugs. He shook his head 'no'.

"What do you want for the pain?" I asked. We don't normally offer patients a choice, but Kent was a colleague so this was a little different.

"Something that works," he groaned.

"Well, do you want it IV or a pill?" I asked. He actually got even paler at the mention of an IV.

"A pill is fine," he said hastily. I tried not to smile. Apparently, the big tough fireman was afraid of needles.

"Ok, I'll be right back," I said and walked out to the desk. Dr. Wallace was on the phone, but it looked like he was on hold, from the way he was drumming his fingers impatiently.

I gestured to ask him if he was on hold, and he nodded. "Kent needs Lortab for pain and an x-ray of his arm. Is that okay?" I asked him. He knew me well enough to know that I had asked about medication allergies already, and he nodded in agreement.

I went to the medication room immediately to get the Lortab first. The sooner I got drugs in Kent, the better. I got the pills and a glass of water and walked back in the room where Jake had raised the head of the gurney up so Kent could swallow. I handed him the pills and held the water glass where he could grab it with his good hand.

He tossed the pills back and then chugged the water, as if he couldn't get the pain medicine in him quick enough. He laid back against the gurney, looking exhausted from the effort.

"They'll be here in a little bit to take an x-ray," I told him and he nodded. Out of habit, I turned and asked Jake if he needed anything. He just shook his head.

"Thanks for all you've done," he said, gratefully. "I'm glad you're on today."

I knew this time he wasn't flirting, and I felt a rush of pride that Jake thought I was a good nurse. That comment from someone as skilled as Jake was high praise, indeed.

Chapter Six

The helicopter had landed and the Life Flight crew was loading up our two patients. I hadn't realized they had a helicopter that could take two people at one time, but I was glad they did. The neighbor had driven to the ER and she was going to take Timmy home with her for now. Apparently, he knew her well, because he was very excited to see her when she got there and he was much calmer, even as they were loading his parents on to the helicopter. He watched, fascinated, and she just stood there with her arms wrapped around him. I was extremely grateful she was there.

Kent's pills had kicked in enough that he could move the arm to get an x-ray. Dr. Wallace hadn't looked at it yet, but that could wait until our patients were safely on their way. The flight crew stopped by the desk to thank us for all our work. They gave us some pens with their logo on them and then strode out the door with the gurneys in tow. Neither one of the patients had ever regained consciousness, and their prognosis was poor. We were all a little somber, as we watched them get wheeled away. This job was supposed to involve saving lives and it was a little tough to swallow when it didn't work out that way.

The neighbor left with Timmy, who waved good-bye to us enthusiastically. I wondered what would happen to him.

"Poor kid," a voice broke in to my thoughts. Jake had wandered out to the desk, now that Kent was feeling a little better. "I wonder what will happen to him," he said.

"I was just thinking the exact same thing," I sighed. "This is so sad."

We both just stood there in silence for a minute. Sometimes there are no words to be said.

Jake ran his hands over his face, suddenly looking exhausted.

"What do you think happened with the fire?" I asked. Of course, there would be an official investigation, but usually the firemen could piece together what had gone wrong.

"Old trailer, and they were using a space heater next to some curtains," he replied. "Timmy was in the other end of the trailer, screaming, when we got there. I think he saw the fire start and didn't know what to do, so he just ran away. The parents were sleeping in that end, and I don't think they ever woke up."

I nodded as I listened. It was such a sad situation that I didn't really know what to say.

"We were taking them out the back door to the ambulance," Jake continued, "because the front door was blocked by flames. Kent turned back to shut the back door, just to cut down on the draft. I was twenty feet away and I heard the tank go. Felt it too, and out of the corner of my eye, I saw Kent go to the ground and just lay there."

He took a long, ragged breath. "I didn't even know what to do first. I still had the lady on the gurney, and all I wanted to do was go make sure my partner wasn't dead." His voice broke on that last word, and he shook his head softly, staring in to space.

Now I really didn't know what to say. Firemen were usually so macho, it was disconcerting to see him let his guard down like that. I reached out and put my hand on his arm. Times like that, a touch can say what words can't.

Jake looked down at my hand and then looked up at me and smiled a little. "Sorry to get so sappy on you," he half-joked, trying to regain his machismo.

"I think the situation calls for it," I reassured him. "Kent's lucky to have you watching out for him."

"Well, I should have noticed the grill before," he said, shaking his head. "But I don't know what we would have done different. It was just a messed up situation and I'm glad it didn't turn out worse than it did."

I nodded in agreement. Even if Kent's arm was broken, he still didn't get off too bad, all things considered. Unfortunately, the people in the trailer weren't as lucky.

Dr. Wallace had finally looked at Kent's x-ray, and the arm wasn't broken, just badly bruised. Kent was half-asleep on the gurney, now that his meds had kicked in, but he woke up enough to hear the doctor tell him the good news. The fire chief had just arrived at the ER after finishing up at the fire and he went in to see Kent.

"Nice way to get a day off." Chief Gregory strode in the room, scowling sternly. He was well over six feet tall with broad shoulders and graying hair, and an intimidating presence in any situation. He glanced over at me and winked slyly. Chief Gregory wasn't nearly as intimidating as he looked, but he liked to have fun with it. I was happy to play along, just to bring a little humor to the room.

"Oh, he'll be able to go back to work in another thirty minutes," I chirped cheerily. "His arm isn't broken, he'll be just fine."

Kent scowled at me for a moment then swung his head to look at the chief. I could see by his expression that the pain meds were clouding his brain a little. His brow furrowed in confusion, he swung his head back to stare at me again, and finally he realized we were joking.

"Yeah, just give me some more of those pills," he said, dropping his head back onto the pillow. "I'll be good."

We all laughed and the mood in the room lightened up somewhat. Some days, you had to laugh or you were going to cry.

Chief Gregory, Kent and Jake were discussing the details of the fire, so I headed back out to the desk to finish my charting. I suddenly realized I was starving, and now that the adrenaline rush was over, I was actually shaking a little. I went to my locker and grabbed a Power bar to eat while I charted. I never had gotten lunch, just a yogurt and a banana earlier.

I was still working on the charts when Jake came wandering back out to the desk. Since I hate charting, I was always looking for any excuse not to do it, and chatting with Jake was a wonderful excuse.

"What's new in the world of Allie?" Jake asked, leaning over the counter toward me.

"Well, my mom is having knee surgery on Monday," I told him.

"Really?" he replied. "Where's she having that done?"

I filled him in on Dr. Steitler and his outreach surgery site in Madison. He was impressed, as well, that she was able to stay in her hometown for the procedure. I hadn't realized how much of a burden it is to have someone hospitalized away from home until my dad was in Springfield Memorial Hospital for a week. This time around was going to be much simpler and easier.

"So, you're going there for the surgery, huh?" Jake asked, looking nonchalant. He actually just looked really tired, and I wasn't sure he was even hearing half of the conversation. Not that I would blame him, he had been through a lot today. My mom's surgery wasn't really that big of a deal compared to being in an explosion.

"She asked me to," I replied. "I wanted to, anyway, but since she asked, I really want to go."

"Good, she'll have someone to watch out for her," he said, grinning. I laughed, but I really hoped we didn't have a repeat of what happened last time. My dad had complications after his surgery and I couldn't get the nurses and doctors to listen to me when I tried to tell them something was wrong. He finally got good care, but that was after I blew up and yelled at a surgeon in the middle of the ICU.

No, this time, things were going to be much different. Mom had an excellent surgeon, and the hometown crew at the hospital were going to give her the royal treatment. I was barely even worried about this surgery. Barely.

"Triage," I heard Tracy call out. I sighed, looking down at my still unfinished charting. That's what I get for socializing.

"I'll let you get back to work," Jake said, turning to walk back into Kent's room. "Tell your mom I said hi and good luck."

I nodded and walked up to the triage window. A young man, about twenty-two was sitting there, in a dirty, oversized t-shirt and baggy shorts. He was what the polite folk called 'husky' and what the medical folk called 'obese'. It always made me sad to see people so young already in such bad shape.

"How can we help you?" I asked him. I knew he wasn't here for help with his weight, so he didn't want to hear about all the problems it would cause him.

"I got a rash," he said, around a wad of gum.

"And where is the rash at?" I asked. The usual questions- where, when, how long, how bad, etc.

He stood up out of the chair and reached down to the elastic waistband on his shorts. I realized with horror that he wasn't going to tell me where the rash was, he was about to show me.

"No, no!" I cried out. "Leave your pants on!"

This was one of those times that my mouth said stuff before my brain had totally processed it. I heard enough noise at the nurses' station behind me to know that everyone had heard me. Fortunately, the young man didn't seem the least bit fazed and just shrugged and sat back down.

"How about we just get you checked in and into a room?" I continued politely. "Then we can finish the questions."

Tracy looked like she was going to choke on her own tongue, but she managed to ask him for his name and date of birth without bursting into laughter. I walked back to the nurses' desk, pointedly ignoring my chortling coworkers. Being single had left me as the butt of many a joke in this department, especially when an 'interesting' male patient came in.

Scott grinned gleefully, and cracked, "Maybe you coulda got a date!" I just smiled and went back to my charting. Might as well finish it up because it seemed we weren't going to slow down any. I really wanted some lunch and some coffee, but it didn't look like that was going to happen.

I finished my chart and added it to the growing stack in the cubby of completed charts. I grabbed the clipboard for young man with the rash and headed for his room. Linda was already up at the triage window, talking to the next arrival.

The young man, Ricky Scott, didn't have much for a health history, so we got through the questions quickly. He had changed in to a gown, and his not-so-clean clothes were piled on the floor. He didn't look or smell like hygiene was too much of a priority for him, and I was a little nervous to see this rash.

I used the blanket to keep as much of him covered as possible as I looked at where he was complaining of a rash. Just as I suspected, it was in his groin folds, and looked like a combination of dirt and sweat that was irritating the skin. Nothing looked contagious or too serious, but I would let Dr. Wallace make the final call on that. I got some warm washcloths and gently washed the area and dried it off really well.

As I was washing my hands, I wondered if Dr. Wallace's good mood was still intact. He had a history of being really blunt with patients like this. It took quite a bit of tact to tell someone that he's just dirty without offending him, and tact was not something Dr. Wallace had much of.

"Chest pain," Tracy called out, and Scott grabbed a wheelchair and headed for the front door. I walked in to the cardiac room and turned the monitor on. Scott wheeled the patient in, a man who looked about forty years old, and no less than three hundred pounds. His round face was red and sweaty, and he was holding one hand over his chest.

He certainly was high risk for heart disease, so this could be a serious situation. Scott helped him get over to the gurney and pulled his t-shirt off. I got the cardiac monitor attached while Scott grabbed the stuff to start an IV.

I asked him the questions as we worked, since time was of the essence in this situation. His name was Alan Merona, and he was forty-two years old. He had never had any problems with his heart, but he did have high blood pressure and type 2 diabetes. He had been eating at Joe's and about the time he finished his burger, he started to feel this intense pressure. His wife drove him straight to the ER, because her father had died from a heart attack, and she wasn't taking any chances.

Scott had a challenge finding a vein with all the extra padding Alan had, but Scott was always up for a challenge. He got the IV in just above Alan's wrist, and drew the blood to send off to lab. I never ceased to be amazed at the stuff Scott could do.

The cardiac monitor didn't show any changes that would indicate a heart attack, but we always confirmed it with a lab test. Dr. Wallace had walked in and asked the patient a few brief questions, then gave me some orders. There was a protocol to follow for chest pain patients, so we all knew what to do.

Because Alan's symptoms started right after he ate, Dr. Wallace also ordered a GI cocktail, which is a little concoction we use to differentiate cardiac pain from gastric upset. It isn't an actual cocktail, just a mixture of liquid medications that effectively eliminate any stomach issues that are mimicking cardiac pain. If the patient still has the pain after they drink it, then we know it's cardiac pain.

I mixed the ingredients together in a cup. The mixture is thick and mint-flavored, thanks to the liquid antacid in it. I've tried a taste of it, and it wasn't terrible, but it wasn't great either. I took it in to Alan and explained that he needed to drink all of it.

He nodded and took the cup from me. He was still red and sweaty and any kind of movement seemed to make him short of breath. He drank the entire cup of medicine at one time and handed the cup back to me, making a face as he swallowed the last of it.

"Blech! That's nasty," he said, shaking his head. I gave him a drink of water to get the taste out of his mouth. His wife was sitting in a chair off to the side of the room, watching him. She looked a little tense, which seemed fitting for the situation, but she didn't say much.

I jotted down some vital signs on the chart and started to explain to Alan that we were waiting for a lab value to see if he had any heart damage. Partway through my explanation, Alan made an urping motion and put his hand back on his chest. His brow furrowed and my heart sank for a moment. Then, he let out the loudest and longest belch I have ever heard. I swore it came with shock waves.

Alan sat there for a moment, then looked up at me, surprised, and said, "Wow! I feel better!"

I just stood there and stared at him for a minute. Finally I asked, "Are you having any pain at all?"

"Nope," he replied, glibly. "Feel great."

"No chest pressure at all?" I asked again, just to be sure. In reply, he belched again, although less impressively this time.

"Nope, I'm right as rain," he said, cheerily. "That little drink really worked!"

I explained to Alan that we still needed to complete the testing to check for a heart attack.

"Why?" he asked. "I feel fine. I'll just be on my way."

"We have to be 100% sure," I replied. "We can't take any chances."

"But I feel better," he argued. "It was just my stomach, not my heart. Besides, I'm a young healthy guy!"

Hoo-boy. Alan was anything but healthy, in fact, he was a major risk for heart disease. It may have been indigestion this go-round, but it was only a matter of time before he did have a heart attack.

"Alan, you have more than one risk factor for heart disease," I started out carefully.

“I do?” he asked, looking genuinely perplexed. “Like what?”

I couldn’t believe that no doctor had ever talked to Alan about his health or his weight. He was forty-two years old and already on high blood pressure medication. Surely his doctor had explained to him how serious that was.

But the look on Alan’s round, rosy face told me that either no one had told him, or he hadn’t understood when they did. Now I was in the hot seat, because people don’t usually like hearing this kind of news.

“Well, you have high blood pressure, diabetes, and you’re obese,” I said, as politely and professionally as possible.

“But that doesn’t affect my heart,” he replied, earnestly. Hmmm. This was going to take more teaching than I could squeeze in to the ten minutes I had.

“Let me get you some printed information,” I told Alan. “I’ll be right back with it.”

We had a collection of handouts about the more common diseases that we could send home with patients. They don’t really hear much of what we say in the ER, so we want them to have something they could look back through when they got home. I found a handout for each of Alan’s maladies and brought the stack back in to him.

“Here, you can take these home,” I told him. “And we do need to complete the testing, so we need to have you stay for two hours. You can read these while you wait.”

He made a face at hearing he had to stay for two hours. His wife finally spoke up.

"It's fine, he will stay," she said tersely. Alan didn't seem inclined to argue with her, so it looked like I had won the battle.

I went back out to the desk to update Dr. Wallace. I checked the lab readout and it told me what I pretty much already knew.

"First troponin is negative," I reported to Dr. Wallace. "He got complete relief with the GI cocktail."

Dr. Wallace looked a little impatient at that news. "I guess we still need to do the two hour markers, huh?" he said, to no one in particular.

"He is pretty high risk," I responded. Dr. Wallace didn't like people- especially nurses- telling him what he should do, so I just stopped at that and let him come to his own conclusion.

"Yeah, better be sure," he finally agreed. He handed me the clipboard for the young man with the rash. He had written discharge instructions, and I was curious how his conversation with the patient went. He was already on to his next patient, though, so I didn't have time to ask. I took the papers and headed in to the room.

"Hey, Ricky," I said as I came through the door. Ricky was sitting on the edge of the gurney, dressed in his own clothes again. I reviewed the discharge instructions with him, which basically said 'Wash with soap, dry thoroughly, keep clean and dry'. Not really the kind of stuff you would expect to see in the ER, but we saw it fairly often. People didn't have a primary care doctor, so they came to us.

Ricky seemed to be in a good mood, so Dr. Wallace must not have said anything too offensive. He thanked me for everything and walked back out the front door of the ER.

"Did you get a number?" Scott whispered to me as he walked past. I tried to whack him with the clipboard but he was too quick for me.

The rest of the shift went by quickly but nothing too exciting happened. I was exhausted and hungry and very happy to see the next shift show up. I gave report on the two patients I still had and headed out the door.

I started my car and was glad that the windshield was clear. I didn't want to be outside scraping windows, but after today, I wasn't going to rely on the defroster any more. I drove home, noting that traffic seemed pretty light for a Saturday night. Maybe everyone was staying home with the cold weather. I certainly didn't have any plans to go anywhere.

The next morning was still cold, but no snow, and just a few clouds. I still bundled up in a turtleneck sweater and boots for church. Our pastor liked to keep the church a crisp sixty degrees, or at least that was how it felt to me. I think he wanted to make sure people stayed awake.

The sermon today was on trusting God and not worrying, which was a good reminder for me. I kept telling everyone that I wasn't even worried about mom's surgery, but I was just kidding myself. I worried about everything, and when things didn't go according to my plan, I struggled with trusting God. I didn't know if the pastor knew how much I needed that sermon today, but I was glad he preached it. Now I just had to follow it.

Shelby and Wade sat with me, which kind of made me feel like a third wheel. I was happy that Shelby found a good guy, but it made me even more aware that I was alone. I knew it was silly to feel that way, but somehow I couldn't help it.

Some of the church ladies always had coffee and baked goods set out after the service, and people hung around and visited. I tried to socialize away from the counter, so I wouldn't be tempted by the pastries. However, Mary Fisher didn't let me get away with it today.

"I made some caramel rolls with your mama's recipe," she told me proudly. "Go try 'em and tell me if they're as good as hers."

Well, I always do what I'm told. I dutifully scooped up a warm, gooey roll and Shelby got one as well. Wade didn't have a basis for comparison, but he took one anyway. They looked and smelled great, and it turned out, they tasted great too.

I nodded my approval as I was still trying to chew the enormous bite I took. I showed Mary a 'thumbs up' with my fingers covered with gooey caramel. Mary made some pretty fantastic rolls. I couldn't say they were better than mom's, just out of loyalty. However, I was willing to say they were just as good, which was enough for Mary. She beamed with pride when we all gave her our approval.

A belly full of warm bread is a great sedative and I was now ready for a nap. The cup of coffee I had with the roll hadn't negated the effect. I got my coat and started working toward the door. Mary and a few others that knew my mom had all sent well wishes her way. I said good-bye to Shelby and told her I would call her when I got to Madison. She and Wade walked toward his car, holding hands. They really were a cute couple.

I sighed and walked to my car, alone. I drove home and walked into my quiet little house. Maybe there wasn't anyone there with me, but that meant I could have the couch all to myself. And I got to pick the TV channel. Not that it mattered what I picked, because fifteen minutes later, I was sound asleep.

I woke up after an hour and went in search of something more nutritious to eat. My fridge was pretty bare, since I was about to leave town for two days. I ate peanut butter toast and an apple. I wasn't super hungry yet, that caramel roll had really filled me up.

It wouldn't take too long to get to my parents. Madison was 45 miles away, but it was a winding two-lane road. Even with allowing extra time for bad weather, it would only take a little over an hour to get there. I didn't need to leave until this evening, but I was starting feel antsy.

I pulled on a sweatshirt and ran over to the neighbors' house. Cathy liked to know when I was going out of town, so she wouldn't worry about me. Besides that, she picked up my mail for me. I let her know what was going on and when I would be back. She told me to drive safe and wished my mom well.

I packed an overnight bag, trying to decide what I wanted to wear for the next two days. I thought about going for comfort and just wearing sweat pants, but what if there was a good-looking doctor? I compromised and packed jeans and cute t-shirts. Relaxed and comfortable, but still attractive. I wasn't an old maid yet.

I finally ran out of busy work to do, and decided to just leave. I didn't want to be driving after dark, I rationalized. I called mom to tell her I was leaving, mostly because I knew she would be mad at me if I just showed up.

The drive was uneventful, thankfully. The roads were dry and the sun was peeking through the clouds. The view wasn't all that scenic- the frost had killed off all the trees and grass, but there was no snow cover yet. Shades of gray and brown covered the landscape.

I pulled into the driveway as the sun was setting. I didn't like this time of year, the sun went down so early. My parents had lived in this house for almost thirty years, so it always felt like coming home again. They had turned mine and Shelby's room into the guest room, so I even got to sleep in the same room as when I was in high school.

My parents' golden retriever, Lady, came sauntering out to meet me, tail wagging, and I petted her soft, silky head. Lady was just about the best dog I've ever known. My parents got her from the pound after Shelby left home and the house seemed too quiet. Why anyone ever got rid of Lady was beyond me. I liked her ten times better than my sister's dog, who was always slobbering on me and insisting I pet her.

Mom met me at the door with a warm hug. "I'm glad you're here," she said, like she always did, although I think she meant it a little more earnestly this time. I was happy that she had asked me to be here for surgery. I knew it was a tough transition for them to go from being the caregiver to being the one needing cared for. Parents and their children all went through this phase as the parents aged, but I didn't think it would start so early for us. My parents were barely in their sixties.

I carried my bags down the hall to my old room, savoring the smell of whatever mom had cooking in the oven. This was her 'last meal' before her surgery, so I hoped she had picked something good. Not that mom ever made anything that was bad. I was suddenly starving at the smell of real food, and I couldn't wait to get to the supper table.

I liked to cook well enough, but making a whole meal for one person was just more trouble than it was worth most days. Then I had to eat the leftovers for the next three days, at which point I was completely sick of that meal. I loved coming to mom's house and getting a home cooked meal.

I wasn't thrilled about the reason I had to be at mom's house, but I was going to enjoy the cooking while I was here.

Chapter Seven

I woke up thirty minutes before the alarm the next morning. I knew there was no way I was going to fall back asleep, but I didn't want to get up and make noise, since my parents were sleeping. I laid there, talking to God, asking him to help mom through the surgery. Then I realized I should probably ask for a little help for myself, because I was getting nervous. I kept telling myself it was a routine surgery. It wasn't doing much to keep me from worrying.

I finally got up and crept down the hall to the bathroom. Then I walked quietly in to the kitchen, and almost yelped when I saw my mom sitting at the table. She smiled at me, but she looked tired.

"Hey mom," I said. "What are you doing up so early?"

"Oh, I just couldn't sleep," she said. Maybe she was a little nervous too. Even with everyone saying how routine and low risk the procedure was, it still had to be nerve-wracking to go under the knife.

I slid into one of the other chairs. I really wanted to make some toast and coffee, but mom wasn't allowed to eat or drink anything and I thought it would be mean to eat in front of her.

"Are you ready for today?" I asked. It sounded like a dumb question, but I didn't know what else to say.

She took a deep breath and then sighed. "I guess," she said. "I just really want it to be over with so I can start to feel better again."

That was understandable. Once her knee was feeling better and she got some more red blood cells made, she would be feeling much perkier. I was glad we were able to get the surgery done so soon.

"Is dad still asleep?" I asked.

"Yes," she replied. "He's always been such a sound sleeper. I wish I could do that."

I agreed. I was a light sleeper, like my mom, and it could be frustrating.

"I'm glad you're going to be here with him while I'm in surgery," mom said. "I know he acts like he's not worried, but he is nervous about me being in the hospital overnight."

I could understand dad's trepidation. Our family hadn't had good luck with hospitals so far. Granted, we hadn't spent much time in them, so it was unfair to judge all hospitals based on that one experience.

"Well, we can keep each other from going stir crazy," I told her. She just smiled at that.

Dad walked in the kitchen just then, looking rested and ready for the day. Mom and I both looked like death warmed over. I guess a good night's sleep does make a difference. Too bad I couldn't just shut my brain off and go to sleep.

We decided to all get dressed and head to the hospital. We were only twenty minutes ahead of schedule anyway.

We drove to the hospital in nervous silence. Dad dropped us off at the front door of the hospital and went to park the car. It was cold this morning, with a skiff of snow on the ground. Winter was definitely setting in.

Mom checked in at the front desk and they handed her some papers to fill out. We sat in the small waiting area and mom answered a hundred medical questions while I stared at a poster of a wildflower. Dad joined us after a few minutes. Mom was the first case of the day, so the hospital was still pretty quiet. We sat there for fifteen minutes, making small talk and waiting for the nurse to come get mom for pre-op.

A lady with round apple cheeks and brown hair up in a ponytail stuck her head inside the room, and asked, "Betty Sanford?"

"Right here," mom said. We were the only people in there, but the rules say to make sure you have the right person. She walked in to the room and smiled. She had a really nice smile with cute dimples that sank into her apple cheeks. I was happy to see a smile. I always felt better when the nurse smiled.

"I'm Bobbi, the pre-op nurse," she introduced herself. She shook mom's hand and then looked at me and dad.

"This is my husband, Bob, and my daughter, Allie," mom introduced us. "She's a nurse in Brighton."

Bobbi grinned at that. "Well, I better keep on my toes then, huh?" she joked. I was relieved to hear her joke about it. Mom always wanted to tell everyone I was a nurse, but sometimes it could make them nervous that they were being critiqued.

Bobbi took mom into the pre-op area to get ready. She told us that she would be back to get us in a few minutes, once mom was changed, and we could hang out with her in her pre-op room.

Mom walked out the door with Bobbi and my heart flipped over in my chest. I told myself I was being ridiculous. She was going to get dressed in a gown and get an IV put in. There was nothing serious happening in pre-op.

Dad and I sat in the silent waiting room as the minutes slowly ticked by. I was really wondering where I could get a cup of coffee, but I decided I should suffer in solidarity with mom. Well, at least until she went into surgery. Then I was going for coffee and breakfast.

Bobbi came back to get us and we walked down a short hallway into a large, brightly lit area. There were six small rooms, all facing out to a nurses' desk. Mom was in one of the rooms, lying on the gurney in a gown. Under the fluorescent light, she looked terribly pale.

"We'll get the IV here in a bit," Bobbi said. "You can just hang out for now."

I pulled the chair up next to the bed and pointed dad to it. He took a seat and reached out to take mom's hand; she smiled at him weakly and squeezed his hand. I leaned against the wall and looked around the room curiously. I had never been in a pre-op area, even in my own hospital. There wasn't much to it. A cart, small table, one chair and a cardiac monitor mounted in the corner. There was a small closet for clothes and a sink in the corner to wash your hands. A curtain hung across the front of the room, providing privacy from the desk outside. I could still hear everything that was going on out there, so I don't know how much privacy it provided.

My phone chirped with a text message, which reminded me that I hadn't turned my phone ringer off when we came in. I looked at the screen and saw it was Shelby, asking what was going on. I shot a text back telling her we were still in pre-op and then turned it to vibrate. I couldn't believe Shelby was awake at 7 o'clock in the morning.

"Do you have any questions, mom?" I asked. I felt responsible for making sure she understood everything that was going on, even though she had a nurse who was perfectly capable of doing it. That pesky nurse switch just would not switch off.

"I don't think so, sweetie," she replied. "Bobbi explained what was going to happen while I was in there."

That was good, because I didn't actually know what went on in there. I knew you had to have a good IV, you couldn't keep any of your own clothes and you had to have your hair covered- all part of the infection control in the OR. That was the extent of my involvement with surgery patients that came through the ER.

Mom was having spinal anesthesia instead of general anesthesia, which meant she wouldn't have to have the breathing tube put in. I knew they gave drugs to sedate her, but I wasn't even sure what they were. It's funny in medicine how each department is so individualized and specialized. I knew all about the ER, but as soon as I left my own department, I was almost as lost as the patients.

I was nervous enough being out of my home element- patients must be petrified. Bobbi had done a great job at putting my mom at ease, because she was resting quietly and looked calm. I felt like climbing the walls.

Bobbi came back in with a small plastic tray with a handle on it and all kinds of stuff in it. I recognized it as the IV start tray, so I gestured to dad to move away from mom. Bobbi smiled and moved in to the chair vacated by dad.

"Ok, Betty, we'll get that IV in now," Bobbi said. She put the tourniquet on mom's arm and found a vein right away. She got the IV without difficulty and taped the tubing in place. She connected a bag of IV fluid and hung it on the hook at the top of the gurney.

"You were an easy one," Bobbi said, smiling down at mom. "I didn't even have to work at that!"

Mom laughed. She had never had an IV before that I knew of, but she did donate blood and they always told her how easy she was to stick. All those years of working outdoors had built up some nice, healthy vessels. They loved to see her come in.

"About ten more minutes," Bobbi told us, and then stepped out of the room. The unit was starting to get busier, as more patients came in. I tried really hard not to peek at the other rooms, even though the curiosity was killing me. What kind of people were in here having surgery today? How many of them were cases of Dr. Steitler's? It sounded like he did several cases on the day he was here.

The curtain was pulled but it didn't do anything to block out sound. I could hear Bobbi trying for an IV in another room, and not having as much luck. The patient was not being very quiet, either.

That was always a tough situation. Having a patient who was a difficult stick was hard enough, and then when they were yelling at you, it didn't make it any easier to hit the vein. Bobbi kept apologizing for having to poke her, but the lady wasn't pacified. I think everyone in the whole pre-op area could hear her yelling and swearing.

A nurse pulled the curtain back just a few inches and asked "Betty Sanford?" When mom replied that she was, he opened the curtain a little farther and walked in. He was wearing the all-blue OR scrubs and had a hair cover and shoe covers on. He looked about fifty, with tan skin and a trim, athletic body. He smiled at all of us.

"I'm David, I'm from the OR team," he said. "I'm here to get you for your knee operation."

"Oh, okay," mom said. She suddenly looked nervous again. Dad squeezed her hand and leaned down to give her a kiss.

"Do any of you have any questions, before we go?" David asked.

"How long will she be gone?" I asked.

"It will be close to two hours total," David replied. "Surgery takes about 45 minutes and then recovery is an hour. Then we'll move her to her hospital room and you can see her then."

I nodded. I couldn't think of anything else to ask and dad didn't look like he had any questions. I walked over to give mom a hug.

"Good luck in there," I said to her, feeling silly as I said it. I had absolutely no idea what you were supposed to say at a time like this. I didn't actually want to rely on luck to get mom through surgery. She was going to be asleep for the procedure, so it wasn't like she had any impact on the outcome.

"Dr. Steitler will come out to the surgery waiting room in about an hour to tell you how the surgery went," David told us. "But if you need to go somewhere and you aren't there, he'll just catch up with you later today. It's usually a pretty boring report," he grinned. "These knee procedures are fairly simple. No excitement at all."

I laughed nervously. "That's just fine with us! We don't care for excitement much in the hospital."

David laughed too, and pulled mom's gurney out of the room. Mom waved at both of us and then they wheeled her down the hall. My heart did a little flip again. I did a good job of looking cool, calm and collected, though. If dad knew I was nervous, he would get nervous too. He seemed to be unfazed by all this, but maybe he was bluffing just like I was.

But standing there watching my mom get wheeled through the double doors at the end of the hall, I suddenly felt like crying.

Dad and I walked back down the hallway to the surgery waiting room, where David had told us to wait. It was a small room, with a few chairs and one small couch. There was a table with a handful of magazines stacked on it, as well as some informational pamphlets from the hospital. This waiting room was very different from the one in Springfield where dad had open heart surgery. That's ok, they can keep their fancy waiting room. I was happy to be here in Madison, where my parents were at home and no one was in serious condition.

Unsure exactly what to do, we sat down in two of the chairs. The TV on the wall was turned on to one of the talking heads news channels. The sound was turned down but it looked like a chunky older man and a young woman in a low cut top were arguing about something. Some economic crisis and whose fault it was, as near as I could tell. The woman had a lot of makeup on, but it wasn't making her look any older.

We had almost two hours before we would get to see mom again, and nothing to do to pass the time. The TV screen flashed to a commercial for a restaurant and I suddenly remembered I was hungry.

"Hey dad, do you want to grab some breakfast?" I asked. He was up for that so we walked down to the cafeteria. For being a hospital, they didn't have much that was healthy. I got some scrambled eggs, a banana and coffee.

A year ago, dad would have gone for the bacon and toast with lots of butter. But he was a changed man, and he got the same thing I did.

We sat at a small table and ate. As we were sipping our coffee, one of dad's friends walked in.

"Hey Bob, how are ya?" he boomed as he walked over to shake dad's hand.

"Howdy, Leroy," dad replied. "What're you up to?"

"Oh, Elaine is gettin' carved up on her knee today," Leroy replied. "You?"

"Betty's havin' the same thing," dad said.

"I guess this fella comes down from Marbleton and does it," Leroy said. "Some fancy knee doctor they got up there."

"Yep," dad nodded. "Makes it easier, not havin' to travel.

"That's for sure," Leroy agreed. "I know they got all the fancy stuff at their big hospital but as long as we got what we need here, might as well do it here. Besides, not too much that can go wrong with a little knee surgery."

Dad and I agreed. That was basically the same discussion we had with Dr. Lytle when we decided to have the surgery done here.

"Leroy, this is our daughter, Allison," dad said, gesturing to me. I reached up to shake his hand.

"Oh, you're the nurse, huh?" Leroy asked. Apparently my dad had talked about me to him before.

"I hear you're pretty good at what you do," Leroy continued, with a grin. I think I actually blushed. It was flattering to know my dad had been bragging about me. My parents were always telling me that they were proud of me, but I figured parents were required to say that. Just like telling you that you were pretty and it was okay that you weren't married yet.

"Well, I do my best," I demurred. I wasn't quite sure how to respond, but I could feel myself still smiling.

"I better get up to Elaine's room," Leroy said. "She goes in to the OR in just a bit." He said goodbye to both of us and walked off. His wife must have been second on the list for the day. I was glad mom was able to get the first time slot of the day. The sooner we got this over with, the sooner I could stop worrying.

We finished up our breakfast and wandered back to the waiting room. Someone had changed the TV channel to a show about antique cars, so dad was entertained by that. I got out my phone and sent texts to Shelby and Andrew that mom was in surgery.

I looked around the waiting room at the other people there. I usually liked to make up stories in my head about people around me. But I was pretty sure everybody's story here was they had a family member in surgery so I couldn't entertain myself with that. There was an older man sitting in the corner, with his head tipped back against the wall and his eyes closed. Every so often, he would snore, then snort and reposition his head. My neck hurt just watching him sleep like that.

A woman in her thirties had her hands full with two kids. The older boy was about ten and it didn't seem he got much discipline. The younger boy was only two, and he was toddling around and getting in to everything. The older boy didn't like having his mom's attention pulled away from him by his little brother, so he was doing his best to keep her focus on him. Unfortunately, his method of choice was a tantrum. She was trying to get him to play a game on his video player. He responded by throwing the player on the floor. About then, the little one knocked a plant over.

The mom jumped up to clean up that mess and the older boy walked over to the table of magazines and shoved them all onto the floor. The two-year-old started running across the room, and the mom looked like she wanted to disappear into the floor. Or break down crying.

I couldn't sit by and watch her struggle like that. It was stressful enough to worry about my mom in surgery. At least I didn't have to worry about anything else at the same time. I grabbed the two-year-old just before he barreled into an elderly lady with a walker and swooped him up in the air, playfully. I really hoped he would think this was fun, or I was about to have a screaming toddler on my hands.

Luck was with me, and the raucous little boy squealed with delight. He didn't seem the least bit concerned that a total stranger was holding him, and his mom didn't seem worried either. That's a nice thing about small towns. Everyone trusts each other. Besides, no one in their right mind would kidnap that kid. He looked like a handful.

I was flying the boy around the room like an airplane, giving his mom a break to placate the older boy. By the looks of the two boys, they didn't have the same dad, which would explain some of the animosity. The older boy had been used to having mom all to himself for a while, and he didn't like sharing her with the new family. That would be a tough situation.

I was getting dizzy spinning around the tiny little room, so we went out in the hall, still flying like a plane. I was having fun with the kid, swinging him around wildly and making airplane noises. Just as we came to a junction in the hallway, we nearly ran into an EMS crew wheeling a gurney with an older man on it.

I stopped abruptly, and the crew stared at me bemusedly. I blushed and reminded myself that they didn't know me or that I was a nurse. It was still embarrassing to be caught acting like a little kid.

The guy on the gurney moaned, reminding the crew they were in the middle of a patient transfer, and they headed on down the hall. Small hospitals sometimes had to transfer patients to bigger cities, and the ambulance crew was the taxi service. I saw them come into Brighton County Hospital every so often.

The little boy watched, wide-eyed, as they passed by and went down the hall. He probably thought the bed with wheels was pretty neat. I was getting worn out from all the flying and packing around a 20-lb kid, so we headed back to the waiting room.

His older brother had calmed down and was playing his video game. His mom had picked up the plant and the magazines and was now slumped in a chair next to him, looking wiped out. She glanced up at me as we walked back in the room.

"Thanks for your help," she said with a tired smile. "I've got my hands full today."

"No problem," I replied. "I've had some experience with distracting kids. Happy to help."

"Oh, are you a teacher?" she asked.

I stifled a snort. Teachers are amazing people, and they have way more patience than I do. I admire them, but I don't even want to do their job.

"No, I'm an ER nurse," I replied.

"Do you work here?" she asked. I shook my head.

"I live in Brighton," I explained. All smaller hospitals were about the same as far as the ER went, though. We saw a little bit of everything, and that included kids. We didn't have the luxury of being specialized in only one type of patient. We had to know a little bit about all of them.

"Well, you seem to have a knack for handling rambunctious little boys," she smiled wryly. The little boy was toddling around the room looking for stuff to get in to. His mom dug a container of cereal out of her bag and called him to come get a snack. Food is always a good way to keep them quiet for a little while.

I went back and sat next to dad. I needed a distraction myself. I wanted to be here when Dr. Steitler came out to talk to us, so I would just have to sit there, slowly going crazy, until then. I leafed through a *Better Homes & Gardens* from two years ago, without really seeing anything on the pages. I set it back down and picked up a *Guideposts* that was just about as old. I figured a little inspirational reading was a good idea right now.

The page I flipped open to was an article about a woman who had some serious medical problem and ended up in the ICU. The doctors were predicting that she wouldn't live through the night and the family was gathering at her bedside, and that was enough for me. I shut the magazine and set it back down. I'm sure she pulled through, or they wouldn't have put it in *Guideposts*, but I didn't even want to think about the ICU. I took some deep breaths and tried to remember that verse in Matthew about not worrying.

My phone buzzed in my pocket and I jumped six inches in the air. Dad gave me a curious, sideways glance and then went back to his TV show. I guess I was wound a little tight this morning. I pulled my phone out and saw it was a text message from Jake. I tried unsuccessfully to smother the smile that stole onto my face, and hoped dad wasn't looking at me.

'*Been thinking about you. How is mom?*' the text said. I was a little surprised that he remembered surgery was today. When I told him about it on Saturday, he was a little distracted with everything that had happened. I would have understood if he had forgotten, but I was still pleased that he had remembered.

'*In OR now,*' I sent back. I didn't really have any more information for him, and sometimes trying to talk, or text, to Jake made my mind go a little blank.

'*How are you?*' he replied. Jake knew I got nervous with these situations and he had been my sounding board during my dad's hospital stay. I wanted to just say 'good', but he would know it was a lie.

'*I'll be better when she's out*,' I responded. He just sent back a smiley face that put a smile on my face. Sometimes it was nice when people just understood that I was a natural born worrier, and trying to talk me out of worrying was futile. I knew somewhere inside my head that worrying didn't do any good, so I didn't need a lecture from anyone.

I stuck my phone back in my pocket, feeling a little more relaxed. As distractions went, Jake was a pretty good one. I was thinking about finding the bathroom when a tall, broad-shouldered man in blue scrubs walked into the waiting room. He had glasses and a head cover on, and he looked vaguely familiar. I was trying to figure out how I might know him when he looked around the room and asked, "Sanford family?"

Dad waved to him and he started walking toward us. I wondered why I would recognize someone from the OR here, but I was sure I had seen him before. He had dark eyes and a serious expression, which was making me a little nervous.

"Dr. Steitler," he said, reaching out to shake dad's hand, and then mine. Well, that was why he looked familiar. I had seen his picture on the website when I was reading all about his amazing surgical skills. In that picture, he was wearing a suit and tie, and a smile. Now, his dark hair was covered with a blue cap and he was in hospital issue scrubs.

"Everything went great," Dr. Steitler said, calmly. "We cleaned out some scar tissue, not a huge amount, but enough to cause her pain. No real blood loss, vital signs were great, she slept through the whole thing. Should be good to go home in a couple days."

He finished talking and looked from dad to me and back. "Do you have any questions?" he asked.

I was still processing what he had said, because with his grim expression, I was just sure he was coming with bad news. It took a second for me to comprehend that he was telling us that everything went great.

"Um, no, I don't," I stammered. "Do you, dad?"

Dad just shook his head and said, "Thanks, doc." Dr. Steitler nodded politely and then turned and walked back out of the room.

I was at a loss for what to do next. We had over an hour before we could see mom, and I didn't want to spend it sitting in this horrible chair, but I didn't know where else to go.

"Dad, I'm going to get another cup of coffee," I said. "Do you wanna go with me?"

He shook his head, still fixed on the TV. I guess he was comfortable here and now that we didn't have to worry about mom, he was engrossed in some show.

I wandered down the hall and filled a cup with steaming, delicious coffee. I found a table in the corner and sat there to call Shelby and Andrew. I gave them both the same brief update. Surgery went great and we hadn't seen her yet.

I sat there, sipping coffee and watching the people coming through the cafeteria. I was suddenly really tired and I wondered if mom's hospital room would have a recliner like dad's had. It made a handy place to take a little catnap.

The chairs in the waiting room weren't conducive to any kind of relaxing, they were just incredibly uncomfortable. I finished my cup of coffee, hoping the caffeine would give me a little jolt of energy. When you drink as much coffee as I do, you can get a little immune to its effects. Which was a bummer on days like today, when I was a few hours shy on sleep. I sighed, and headed back to the waiting room. I would get a good night's sleep tonight, now that mom was safe and sound.

Only twelve hours until bedtime.

Chapter Eight

I hadn't been back in the waiting room long when Bobbi stuck her head in the door, looked around and smiled when she saw us.

"She's ready to head to her room, if you want to come along with us," she said. Dad and I stood up and grabbed our stuff. Mom had packed a bag, since she knew she was staying a couple of days, and I grabbed that before dad could. It wasn't really heavy, but he wasn't supposed to lift since he had had open heart surgery.

We walked out in the hall and mom was laying there on a gurney, looking a little sleepy but comfortable.

"Hi mom," I said, smiling, and trying to ignore the tears that were threatening to well up in my eyes. "How are you?"

She smiled goofily at me as dad reached over to squeeze her hand. She rolled her head in his direction and smiled even goofier. It looked like my mom was three sheets to the wind. I had given enough sedative drugs to know that a lot of people woke feeling tanked. She would sleep it off in a few hours.

Bobbi pushed the cart down the hall and dad and I walked along beside her. She was telling us how great mom did in recovery and that everything looked good. We had reached the inpatient wing and Bobbi stopped in front of one of the doors.

“This is it,” she said. “Room 134.” She maneuvered the gurney into the room as another person came in the room to help transfer mom over to the bed. Dad and I waited in the hallway until they had mom all situated and Bobbi came back out with the now empty gurney.

“Thanks for everything,” I said to Bobbi. “You were really great with mom.”

“No problem,” Bobbi replied, with a smile. “She’s such a sweetheart. Good luck and it was nice to meet you.” She headed down the hall and dad and I turned to walk in the room.

The lady standing by the bedside was petite with curly brown hair pulled up on top her head. She was wearing a scrub top with Looney Tunes on it, which made me like her instantly.

“Hi, I’m Leah,” she introduced herself, with a smile.

“I’m Allie, her daughter,” I said. Dad just stood there, so I added, “This is Bob, her husband.”

“Nice to meet you,” she replied. “I’m just going to check some vital signs and do an assessment. You can make yourselves comfortable.” She motioned toward the recliner and two other chairs that were sitting off to the side of the room.

The recliner looked nice and comfy, but I had had enough sitting for awhile. I pointed dad toward the chair and then I started unpacking mom’s bag and putting stuff away. She hadn't brought much, so I put her few toiletries in the bathroom and her clothes in the small closet. I set her cell phone and Bible on the bedside table, so she would have them close by when she finally woke up.

Leah finished up what she was doing and gathered up her supplies. She told us she would be back in a few minutes and bustled out the door. I had heard that surgical wings were busy and she didn't look like she gathered much moss.

I walked over to the bed and touched mom's hand gently. She looked up at me blearily. "Allison?" she said, sounding and looking a little confused.

"Mom, you're done with surgery and now you're in your room," I reminded her. "How do you feel?"

She stared at me for a long moment and finally slurred, "I feel jush fine." Then her head lagged back on to the pillow. Looks like mom is a bit of lightweight. I tried not to giggle at the sight. At least she wasn't in pain.

Leah bustled back in the room with some papers and a cup of ice chips. She set everything on the bedside table and then turned to talk to us.

"She's still sleeping off the drugs, so we're just going to let her sleep," she explained. "This machine will check her oxygen level, heart rate and blood pressure automatically, and I'll just keep checking in." She pointed to the ice chips and said, "She can have some of those if she wants, but not until she's more awake. Call me if you need anything."

Dad and I nodded and Leah bustled back out the door. My patience was starting to wear thin. I hadn't done anything but sit all morning and now I got to sit some more. I wasn't one to sit and do nothing. I got too antsy.

I had already had two cups of coffee, so I couldn't really use that as an excuse to move around. In fact, they might be part of why I'm so antsy now.

"Why don't you go find me a paper?" dad said. "It'll give you something to do. Keep you from crawling the walls."

Apparently, I looked as antsy as I felt. I was relieved to have some reason to walk around. I wasn't even sure dad really wanted a newspaper, I think he just wanted to give me something to do. That was fine with me. I grabbed my purse and headed down the hall.

I didn't know the hospital in Madison very well, which gave me an excuse to wander down every hall I found, as I pretended to be looking for the gift shop. I walked past a very serious looking set of double doors with a phone on the wall outside. Right next to it was a window that looked in to the nursery, and the doors had a sign instructing visitors that they had to call for permission to enter. Security was pretty tight around the babies, even in a small hospital. Farther down that hallway was another secured door that said 'Pharmacy'. Looks like they had all the drugs locked up too. Good to know that nobody was going to wander off with a baby or some morphine.

I got to an intersection in the hallway and a sign said 'Gift Shop' with an arrow to the right. However, another sign said 'Emergency' with an arrow to the left, and I decided to wander that direction first. I was just curious to see how their ER looked, even though I wasn't sure I would be able to see it. The ER doors were usually secured as well, more for the staff's safety than the patients'. But I could at least check out their waiting room.

I reached the waiting room near the end of the hallway and peeked in. No one was in there, so I walked in and looked around. It wasn't very big, much like the rest of the hospital. There were some plastic toys stacked in the corner and a few magazines on the one table. The poster on the wall instructed everyone to cover their cough and use the hand sanitizer. The check-in desk was behind a glass window and no one was sitting at it right now. There was doorbell to ring if you needed help, but obviously I didn't, so I turned to walk back out.

As I was headed for the door, a middle aged woman in all white scrubs walked by in the hallway and stopped when she saw me.

"Can I help you?" she asked. Her voice was a mixture of friendly helpfulness and suspicion as to why I was walking around the ER waiting room but not ringing the bell for help. I was familiar with this. Sometimes, people who were up to no good like to loiter in the hospital, hoping for an opportunity to access some drugs. I didn't take it personally, but I was a little embarrassed at getting caught.

"I, um, no," I stammered. I didn't think she would buy the 'looking for the gift shop' line. That would just make me look more suspicious.

She raised an eyebrow at me, and I decided to just come clean.

"My mom had surgery today and I'm going crazy sitting in that room," I confessed. "I'm just walking around to burn off some energy."

She smiled at that and then looked at me a little closer. "Is your mom Betty Sanford?" she asked.

"Yeah," I replied, startled.

"You look like her," the lady said, smiling. "I saw her name on the schedule for today. How is she doing?"

"She's good," I replied. "She's still pretty groggy from the sedation so we're just watching her sleep. The surgery went great."

"It's so nice for people here that Dr. Steitler comes down," she said. "I'm Karen, by the way, the nursing supervisor today."

"Nice to meet you," I said, shaking her hand. "Allie Sanford."

"You're a nurse, aren't you?" she asked.

"Yep, I work in the ER at Brighton County," I replied. Apparently, my mom had talked about me as well.

"I was a terrible daughter when my mom was sick," Karen confided. "I was so stressed and I took it out on the hospital staff. I nitpicked everything they did, and I fired more than one nurse." She shook her head as she recalled that. "I don't know why I did it. I sure didn't make things any better for my mom." She laughed and added, "I hope you didn't do that."

I shook my head emphatically. "No, everyone here has been great!" I gushed. We had only had two nurses so far, but they had both been good. I tried not to nitpick the nurses anyway. I knew firsthand how annoying it was.

"Well, I'll stop in and see Betty in a couple hours," Karen said. "Enjoy your tour of the hospital."

I thanked her and walked back down the hall toward the gift shop. I wished it was nicer weather, so I could go walk around outside and not look suspicious. However, as I passed a window, I saw it was snowing and windy still, so I was stuck indoors.

I got to the gift shop and browsed for awhile. At least it was normal to loiter in a shop. I found dad's newspaper and got a book and some Hot Tamales for me. I thought about getting one of the cute little 'Get Well' stuffed animals, but I was sure mom was going to get a flood of flowers and gifts and she didn't need one more. My parents were well-liked in this town, and in small towns, it seemed everybody knew if you were in the hospital.

I headed back to mom's room with the goods. Dad was kicked back in the recliner, watching TV with the sound turned down low. Mom was still asleep. I took a seat in one of the other chairs and set my purchases on the side table.

I suddenly remembered I hadn't updated my siblings on mom's status, so I dug out my phone and sent a message to both of them that mom was in her room but still sleepy. I hesitated for a moment, wondering if I should text Jake as well. Then I decided to stop overthinking it and sent him a message. He had asked how she was, it made perfect sense to send him an update.

Shelby texted back, asking when she should call and talk to mom. I replied that we would call her when mom was more awake. Andrew had about the same question and he got the same answer. Shelby had really wanted to come with me, but we had decided that I would come for surgery and then Shelby would come over when mom went home, so she could help out at the house.

My phone buzzed again, and this time it was Jake. '*Glad she's doing good. Hope you're better now, too,*' the message read. I smiled at that. Yes, I was less nervous now that I could see for myself that she was doing fine, and I sent him a message that said that.

I used to wonder why patients' family members insisted on seeing them, even when I had assured them they were doing fine. Usually, the patient was sleeping and all they did was go in and look at him, so I didn't understand why they wouldn't just stay in the waiting room and watch

TV. But now I understood. A hundred people could tell me my mom was fine, but I still needed to see it with my own eyes.

Speaking of eyes, mom's were starting to flutter open, so I walked up to her bedside.

"Mom?" I said softly, as I touched her hand. She opened her eyes, a little more briskly this time, and smiled faintly.

"How are you feeling?" I asked. Her brow furrowed as she contemplated the question and she started to answer, but her mouth was dry and her tongue seemed stuck in place.

"How about some ice chips?" I offered and she nodded. I grabbed the cup and spooned a couple pieces of ice into her mouth. She chewed them up and swallowed them with gusto.

"Oh, those are delightful," she sighed. I offered her another spoonful and she took them eagerly. I had heard patients say that your mouth was horribly dry when you woke up from anesthesia.

Now that mom was able to speak, I asked the more important question, "Are you having any pain?"

"No, not really," she said. "Can I sit up a little bit?"

I used the button on the side rail to raise the head of her bed up and she readjusted herself in the bed. She looked down at her knee curiously, but it was covered with a sheet.

"Can I see what it looks like?" she asked. I was a little curious myself. I pulled back the sheet and was slightly disappointed to see her entire leg covered in a white compression stocking. I guess that made sense, to have TED hose on after surgery. I could make out the outline of two small bandages, on either side of her knee. Well, they did tell us it was minimally invasive, so I guess two little bandages were all she needed. I was just remembering dad having dressings that ran the length of both legs and I could tell that's what mom was thinking too.

"Well, that doesn't look bad at all," she said, sounding relieved. She wiggled her toe and then tried to move her leg, but then stopped and grimaced slightly.

"Does it hurt?" I asked her. I was concerned that she wasn't going to tell us when she had pain and I knew pain control was important so that she would move the knee.

"It's just a little stiff," she replied, gingerly moving the leg a little. The leg and knee were a little swollen compared to the other leg, which would explain some of the stiffness.

Leah walked back in just then and smiled when she saw mom was awake.

"Well, it's good to see your eyeballs," she said cheerfully. "How does the leg feel?"

"Just a little stiff," mom replied. "It doesn't really hurt."

"That's good," Leah said. "There is some swelling there. I need to put this ice pack on the site, I forgot to do that earlier." She carefully placed an ice pack over the knee.

"Dr. Steitler has only done about four of these OR days down here, so I'm still not in the routine of what the patients get," Leah explained. "We never did knee surgery here before."

"Well, you're doing a great job," mom reassured her, and I nodded in agreement. Forgetting an ice pack for an hour was not a major thing.

"I have these other things to put on too," Leah continued. "They're called SCDs and they help prevent blood clots from forming in your legs." She held up a blue cloth device that connected to a pump by a long plastic tube. She lifted up mom's good leg first and wrapped the piece around her calf and fastened the Velcro closure. She carefully repeated the process on the left leg, and mom grimaced slightly with the movement. Leah made sure the ice pack was back in place and then she switched on the pump, which was at the end of the bed.

Mom watched the cuffs, fascinated, as one slowly inflated and then deflated again. Then the other one did the same thing.

"Those help keep the blood moving through your veins until you get up and start walking," Leah explained. "Some people don't mind them, and some people think they're really annoying. Either way, they're really important, so we need to have them on."

Mom didn't seem to mind them much. She reached for her cup of ice chips and ate some more.

"Do you want to try some Jell-O?" Leah asked her. Mom thought that sounded wonderful and Leah said she would be back shortly with some.

Dr. Steitler suddenly walked in, walking straight to mom's bed to look at her knee. Seeming satisfied with what he saw, he then looked up at her and asked her how she was doing. His stern look softened a little, and he even smiled at her.

"I did four knees today, and yours looks the best, Betty," he told her. Maybe he said that to all the patients, but I still liked hearing it.

Mom just smiled and thanked him for his work. He turned and asked dad and I if we had any questions, and we didn't. He nodded in our direction and then turned and walked back out. Not the most congenial guy, but then we weren't paying him for his personality.

Leah came back with the Jell-O, which mom polished off in short order. She had also brought some apple juice and a pitcher of water. Mom was sucking down liquids like we were stranded in a desert. That was good, the more she drank, the sooner she could get rid of her IV fluids.

However, her kidneys were in great shape, so pretty soon, she needed to get up to the bathroom. Of course, she wanted to try to just get up herself, since she wasn't used to needing people to help her. I reminded her that she had a whole bunch of stuff connected to her and we needed Leah's help for that. I pushed the call button for help.

Leah arrived within moments and mom told her she needed to get up to the bathroom.

"Oh good," Leah said. "We can try out that new knee." She smiled at mom, who attempted to smile in return. I was still concerned that mom was hurting and refusing to tell anyone.

Leah disconnected the SCDs on mom's legs and maneuvered the IV pole around so it was on the same side of the bed. She grabbed a walker that had been sitting in the corner and set it by the IV pole. Then she helped mom sit up at the side of the bed.

"Let's just sit for a minute," Leah said to mom.

"Oh no, I'm fine. I can get…." Mom's voice trailed off and she bobbled as she was sitting. Leah steadied her with a firm hand on her shoulder.

After a minute, mom seemed to be recovered. "I've never gotten lightheaded like that," she said, sounding concerned.

"It's normal after surgery," Leah reassured her. "That's why we always make people sit for a minute before they get up."

"Well, I guess I should learn to listen to the nurse," mom said, wryly. I bit my tongue to keep from pointing out that she never listened to me, and I was a nurse. I guess it didn't count when you were also the daughter.

Mom very carefully pulled herself up to a standing position. She grabbed on to the walker, but Leah stopped her again.

"Just stand for a minute," she said gently. Mom was already starting to look pale.

"You can sit back down if you need to," Leah told her. Mom shook her head but didn't say anything. After a few moments, you could see mom clearing up as the blood supply returned to her head. She reached for the walker and gingerly took a few steps. She wasn't really putting any weight down on the left leg, just sort of tip toeing with it. I watched her face for signs that she was having pain but she seemed to be doing really well.

Leah wrangled the IV pump and they made their way into the bathroom without incident. I was relieved to see mom already up and around. It just reaffirmed to me that this would be a quick and easy recovery.

Mom made her way back to bed from the bathroom, and Leah reconnected everything. Mom was actually starting to feel hungry now, and since she hadn't had any nausea with the Jell-O, Leah said she could get something a little more substantial. Mom ordered some chicken noodle soup and apple juice.

“Do you need something?” she asked me and dad. “Did you eat lunch yet?”

Always the mother. She just had surgery but she’s worried that dad and I haven’t eaten. I assured her we were fine and we would go get something in the cafeteria later. I wasn’t really hungry, and dad looked too comfy to move right now. I guess he could relax better in the hospital when he wasn’t the one in the gown.

After mom finished her juice and soup, she decided she had had enough activity for a while and she was going to take a little nap. I took that as our exit cue, and dad and I headed to the cafeteria.

I would have preferred to go somewhere and get lunch, since the cafeteria had such a limited selection, but a glance out the window changed my mind. I’ve gone out in weather worse than this, but I couldn’t justify taking the risk just for lunch.

We got downstairs and I was pleasantly surprised to see baked chicken and vegetables at the entrée counter. I also saw angel food cake at the dessert bar, but it had berries on it, so it was practically healthy. Dad skipped the cake but did get a fresh, still warm dinner roll with butter. He never did have a sweet tooth like I did. Maybe I got it from my mom. Well, we were eating pretty healthy overall, so one little splurge wasn’t going to hurt.

While we ate, I debated whether we needed to stay the rest of the day at the hospital. It felt a little weird not to stay here with mom, but it wasn’t like we were doing anything for her. We were kind of in the way in her hospital room, even though Leah hadn't made us feel that way. I could still tell that moving around in the room was more difficult with us taking up space, and as long as dad was camped out in the recliner, mom would end up staying in the bed.

"Maybe we should go home for a bit and let mom rest," I suggested nonchalantly to dad. "She's doing good and not too much is going to happen for the rest of the day. We could go home and take care of stuff at the house and come back to visit this evening."

Dad just shrugged and said, "I don't mind hanging out here. That recliner is pretty comfy and they have cable."

This wasn't going to be as easy as I had hoped. I knew mom would never make dad get out of the recliner so she could sit in it, but she needed to get up and around. Laying in the bed all day wasn't going to help her recover. I also wanted to get everything ready at the house so she didn't have to worry about any of it when she came home.

"Dad, mom needs to be sitting in the recliner, not you," I pointed out.

"Why can't she just lay in the bed?" dad asked.

"How much did you want to lay in the bed after your surgery?" I asked him, pointedly. He mulled that over and I could tell I had made my point.

"Ok, we'll go home," he said. "Need to feed the dog, anyway."

We decided we would go back up and see how mom was doing, and then go home if everything looked good. Mom was still asleep when we got back to the room, and that qualified as good for me. I caught Leah in the hallway to tell her we were going home for a while and make sure she had our phone number, just in case.

We walked out the front door of the hospital into a strong wind that was driving snow almost sideways. I tucked my face into my jacket and we walked quickly to the car. Dad had to scrape ice off the windows and I sat in the car, wishing it would warm up faster. It felt weird to have someone else scraping the windows while I just sat there. This must be what it was like to have a husband do that stuff for you. I have to admit, right now, it felt pretty nice to sit inside the car while someone else scraped the windows.

Dad carefully drove home and we hurried inside. Lady was happy to see us, but after I petted her, she went back over to her bed and laid back down. She wasn't too interested in going outside, and I didn't blame her for that.

I looked around the kitchen to see what they might need from the grocery store. Mom was the one who took care of the house, including the groceries. I'm sure dad could figure it out if he had to, but I was worried mom would just try to do it, when she was supposed to be taking it easy. I had met a lot of people who had problems after a joint surgery, and when I questioned them, they all had to admit that they hadn't followed their activity restrictions. I wanted mom to follow every single restriction so her knee would heal up right.

Patients were funny like that, sometimes. They wanted to have the surgery work out well, but they didn't want to participate in the process. If I had someone carving on me, I would be following the rules religiously, just so I didn't have to go back under the knife.

I checked my phone and sent text message updates to Andrew and Shelby, and replied to a couple other friends who had asked about my mom. I was stretched out on the couch in the living room and starting to think that a nap sounded like a really good idea.

My phone buzzed again and it was Jake. '*What did the 0 say to the 8?*' his message read. Before I could reply, a second message came in, '*Nice belt.*'

I couldn't help but chuckle at the joke. It was nice to have a little humor sent my way, and I sent a message telling him I appreciated the comic relief.

'*See? I'm more than just a pretty face!*' he replied. That was true, but his pretty face was what he was best known for. Even women who didn't know his name still knew he was the 'hot fireman'. I don't think it bothered him too much to be famous for his looks.

'*And I appreciate all of your attributes,*' I replied. I really did. Jake was funny and compassionate, as well as smart. He was very good at his job and he loved helping people. In spite of being the 'hot fireman', he wasn't really conceited, and for all his flirting, he didn't date much. He certainly could have bounced from girl to girl if he wanted to, and plenty of them made it clear they were interested and available.

Sometimes I wondered why Jake was still single. And I wondered if his mom tried to fix him up with girls because she was worried he would never get married and have a family. Or maybe that was just my mom. I mulled this over as I finally lost my fight with sleep and dozed off.

Chapter Nine

We went back up to visit mom around 7 o'clock that evening. I told dad we wanted to wait until she had a chance to eat supper, but my ulterior motive was to wait until shift change, so I could meet the night shift nurse. That way I could sleep a little easier tonight.

Mom had just gotten back to bed from the recliner when we got there, and dad happily took her place in the chair. She looked pretty good and she said she ate all of her dinner without any trouble. She had agreed to take a pain pill before she got up to the chair and she wasn't having any pain right now.

I was glad to hear she took pain medication. I didn't really think it would be too much of a problem with her, but after all the trouble caused by the ibuprofen she took for knee pain, I was worried she might be hesitant to take anything else. Of course, the pain medication she was getting now was a completely different drug and didn't have the same risk as the ibuprofen did. But most people, my mom included, wouldn't know that.

I remembered a lady from my nursing school clinicals that had had abdominal surgery and adamantly refused to take narcotics. She didn't like how they made her feel, 'all loopy', and no one could convince her that they were necessary, at least for a few days. She was literally writhing in the bed in pain, but still refusing meds. Of course, she had complications from her surgery because she wouldn't get up and walk and wouldn't take deep breaths or cough. She ended up with pneumonia and bowel problems, and spent an extra week in the hospital.

I was horrified at the time that the nurses didn't make her take the morphine, but I learned quickly that it was the patient's right to refuse. Forcing her to take the medication was actually considered battery and could be prosecuted by law. Well, that explained why the nurses had to let her suffer, but it didn't make it any easier to watch.

Mom's bedside table already had a bouquet of flowers, a balloon, a card and a box of candy on it. The church had sent the flowers, and the card and candy were from Karen, the nursing supervisor I had met earlier in the hall. The note in the card told mom to use the chocolates to bribe the nurses, and I had to laugh at that.

We were sitting around chatting when a rotund man in gray scrubs ambled in to the room. He was about thirty-five years old, with brown hair, glasses and a brown goatee decorating his round, friendly face.

"Evenin', y'all," he drawled, smiling his way around the room. "I'm Riley, and I'll be the nurse for the night."

We all said hello to Riley and he ambled over to the bed to check on mom. He was pretty 'fluffy', as they would say in the south, so I imagine ambling was as speedy as his gait got.

"Well, miss Betty, you look too good to be a hospital patient," he flirted with my mom. "You better start looking worse, or I'm gonna have to run you out of here."

Mom smiled at his teasing. I was glad she had a friendly nurse for the night. Night time can be lonely in a hospital and a lot of surgery patients don't sleep much that first night because they were asleep half of the day. At least she would have someone to chat with.

Riley finished checking out mom's leg, and looked around the room.

"Well, Betty, you didn't mention your sister was here!" he gushed, shooting me a wink. Mom actually giggled at that remark, which made me giggle too. Dad just sat there, watching TV, entranced by some guys running around with a ball.

I was satisfied that mom was in good hands for the night. Not only was Riley friendly and funny, but I had watched him as he was assessing mom and he was very thorough.

"Now, miss Betty, you just ring if you need anything," Riley told mom, as he headed out the door. "I'll be back in an hour with some pills."

Mom looked at me, puzzled. "What do I need more pills for?" she asked.

I was sort of guessing, since I didn't know what the doctor had ordered, but I winged it.

"I think you have to take a stool softener so you don't get too constipated from the pain pills," I explained. That was my best guess on what the pills were. There might be an antibiotic, but that would probably be in the IV.

"Oh. I'm not used to taking all these pills," mom sighed. I didn't bother pointing out that so far she had taken exactly one pill, and she was going to take one more, which wasn't really a lot. I guess, if she was used to no pills, two was a lot.

I suddenly remembered that I had promised Shelby and Andrew that I would have mom call them when she woke up. Whoops.

"Uh, mom, have any of the other kids called?" I asked, trying to sound nonchalant.

"Shelby did," mom replied. "It was nice to talk to her. That Wade is such a nice, young man. It sounds like they're getting serious."

There was my mom for you. Shelby called to ask her about her surgery, and instead they ended up talking about Shelby's dating life.

"Andrew and Nicole didn't call?" I asked.

"No, but I'm sure they're busy with the girls," mom brushed it off. She was the least self-centered person I knew. It was amazing. However, Andrew probably hadn't called because I had promised we would call him, and he was very likely worried sick that something was wrong. I pulled out my phone and hit his name.

Andrew answered before the second ring, which confirmed my fears. I jumped right in with the apology.

"I'm super, super sorry, I forgot to call you, she's doing just fine," I rattled off without stopping. There was a long pause on the other end.

"Well, I'm glad she's fine," he replied, carefully. Andrew and I had been in some pretty heated arguments over the years, and I could tell he was trying to keep his cool.

"Here, I'll let you talk to her," I sidestepped the tension by handing my phone over to mom.

Mom chatted with Andrew and filled him in on the events of the day, at least the ones she remembered. I heard her voice get cheerier and I knew Andrew's twin girls, Cassie and Sammie, had gotten on the phone to talk to Nana.

Some kids were scared of the phone and didn't like to talk on it. Not those two. They were going to need their own phone line by the time they got to kindergarten. Mom was trying to talk to one at a time, but they kept fighting over who got the phone. Their mom must have finally stepped in, because I heard mom say, "Oh, hi Nicole."

They chatted for a few more minutes and then mom handed me back the phone. I was about to just stash it in my bag but mom said, "Nicole wants to talk to you."

I swallowed hard and said, “Hi Nicole,” as calmly as possible. Nicole and I got along great, and I was usually happy to talk to her, but I had a bad feeling that right now she was going to tell me how upset Andrew was, which would make me feel like the worst sister ever.

“Hey, Allie,” she said, cheerily. “We were thinking of making a trip out there for the holidays, and I wanted to know which holiday you had to work.”

Oh, well that was an easy question to answer. “I have to work Thanksgiving, and New Year’s Day,” I replied. “I have Christmas Eve and Christmas off.”

“Well, looks like a Christmas trip, then!” she said brightly. “You better have a good tree for Santa to put presents under.”

I heard a commotion in the background when Nicole mentioned Santa. The girls were only three years old last year at Christmas, and I couldn’t believe they remembered who Santa was. They had turned four in July, but they talked and acted more like six. Or thirteen, depending on the day.

I promised to have an incredible tree with lots of space for presents under it, and the girls were pacified with that. Good thing it was less than two months until Christmas, as excited as they were.

Well, now that I had checked out the nurse and updated the family, I figured I was done with my daughter duties for the evening. And I was getting tired really fast. My twenty minute catnap had helped, but I was fading.

Dad saw me yawning and picked up the hint. He turned off the TV, got up out of the recliner and walked over to mom's bedside.

"Now, Betty, you be good," he chided her gently. "And no more flirting with that young man."

He smiled as he said that, and mom smiled back. Dad had seemed like he didn't even notice Riley, but apparently it was just an act. He kissed mom tenderly, and I felt like a third wheel standing there, watching them. Which was getting to be a familiar feeling.

After my parents were done canoodling, I gave mom a hug, told her I loved her and I would see her in the morning. Dad and I headed for home in the chilly November air. It had stopped snowing but there was the ominous feeling that came before a bad storm. It was a sixth sense that was finely tuned if you lived in this area long enough. I prayed I was wrong and the weather would stay clear. I needed to get back to Brighton and Shelby needed to get here, and we didn't need a winter storm messing with our plans.

The road from Brighton to Madison wasn't too bad, and they kept it plowed really well. There was a winding canyon that left Madison heading south, and that road was brutal in bad weather. The local EMS service was volunteer firemen, and they had quite a challenge cleaning up from some of those wrecks. The road wound tightly right next to the river, and people usually drove too fast for conditions. I was thankful I didn't have to drive that road to get home.

We walked in the house and Lady came over to say 'hi'. She rubbed against dad and then me, and then looked past us, like she was looking for someone else. I realized that she was looking for mom, and couldn't understand why she hadn't come home with us. I didn't have any way to tell Lady that mom was just in the hospital and she would be home soon, so poor Lady was going to stay perplexed. She kept looking toward the door and drawing up her eyebrows in confusion.

When dad had his heart attack, the neighbor had come over and gotten Lady to watch her while he was in the hospital. The guy said Lady just laid on the front porch every day, looking down the driveway, morosely. When a car drove past, she would pick her head up to see if it was dad's, but then drop it right back down. A couple times, she even stood up when a car like theirs went by, and he said it was heartbreaking to see her face when she realized it wasn't her 'parents' coming home.

I felt bad for Lady that she was missing mom and I couldn't explain it to her. I got some doggie treats out of the cupboard, but she wasn't interested in eating anything. I sighed and just scratched her ears. There wasn't much else I could do.

Finally, I went to bed, since I was falling asleep on the couch. I made sure my phone was on the charger with the ringer on high. I also checked that the house phone ringer was turned on and the line was working. Just in case.

I snuggled down under my pile of covers and spent some time talking to God. I thanked Him for a successful surgery and good nurses. I asked Him for quick healing and a full recovery and about then I fell asleep. It's a good thing He knew what I was asking for, because I didn't even finish the sentence.

I woke up a little before 7 the next morning. Lady was standing at my bed, with her nose two inches from my face, and I could feel her breath. I opened one eye and looked at her. She didn't seem distressed, just lonely. I rolled over, not really ready to face the day, and Lady whimpered. Guess I wasn't going back to sleep.

I climbed out of bed and stepped into my slippers. They were warm and fuzzy and green plaid. They were incredibly ugly and incredibly comfortable. I got them as a white elephant gift two years ago at the hospital Christmas party. I don't know why I even tried them on to start with, but after I wore them, I didn't want to take them off. Besides, there were no fashion police in my parents' kitchen.

I padded down the hall, thinking Lady needed to be fed or let out, and was surprised to see my dad sitting at the table.

"Morning," I said. "Did you just get up?"

"Nope, been up for a bit," he replied.

"Why is Lady waking me up then?" I asked, puzzled.

"Beats me," dad shrugged. "I already fed her and let her out."

I looked over at Lady, who was laying on her bed, avoiding my gaze and acting innocent. I guess she just thought I needed to get up.

Dad had made a pot of coffee so I filled a cup to drink before I got into the shower. I didn't know my dad even knew how to make coffee, so I was a little surprised to see that he had. Seems my dad had hidden talents I knew nothing about. The coffee was delicious.

I headed back to the bathroom and hopped in the shower. My morning beauty routine didn't take long. It also didn't end with me looking all that beautiful, but I was okay with that. I didn't have the patience to spend an hour getting ready.

My parents had a garage that actually held a car, and it was nice not having to deal with frosted over windows, or a car that was ten degrees inside. Maybe I should add on a garage to my house. We headed for the hospital under the dark gray skies. Tuesday morning in Madison didn't look too lively so far.

When we got to mom's room, she was already sitting up in the chair, with breakfast in front of her. She looked up at us and smiled widely when we walked in.

"Hi mom," I said, reaching down to give her a hug.

"Oh, my! You're cold," she exclaimed. I had forgotten about that. I shucked off my coat and stashed it in the little closet.

"How is breakfast?" I asked conversationally. I doubt the food was amazing, but it looked edible, at least. Dad and I had eaten breakfast at home, since we knew the hospital cafeteria didn't have much to offer.

Mom had some toast and cream of wheat with a cup of tea. She had eaten most of it. I was thinking she needed something with a little more protein to help her heal, but I knew this was what the doctor had ordered for her to eat. She would be home tomorrow, probably, so it wasn't a big deal.

I asked about her night and she said it was uneventful. She slept off and on, and then at 6 o'clock, Riley had helped her get up in the chair. She had taken another pain pill this morning, and was feeling pretty good right now.

I told her Lady was missing her and she smiled sadly. "Poor girl, she's getting tired of us leaving her," she sighed.

"You'll be home in no time and she'll be excited to see you," I reminded mom. She nodded in agreement.

"Did Dr. Lytle come by yet?" I asked.

"Yes, he was here right before I got out of bed," mom replied. "He said everything looks good. He was headed to the office for the day, but said he would stop back this afternoon."

I had heard that surgeons make early rounds, but I didn't realize they were *that* early. I didn't really want to get up at 5 a.m. just to catch the doctor on rounds, so I hoped I got to see him this afternoon. I was mostly wanted to know which day she got to go home. She looked really good, but I didn't know if she could go today, or had to wait until tomorrow.

I walked over to check out her knee, out of curiosity, and it looked about the same to me. She was developing a bruise on the inside of her knee, and she caught me staring at it.

"Dr. Lytle said that's normal," she told me. "It's blood from the inside working its way out and that's why it didn't show up until later. It really doesn't hurt."

I noticed that the blue sleeves on her legs weren't attached to anything.

"Are these supposed to be connected?" I asked her. I could see the plastic tubing laying under the bed.

"Oh, Rachel disconnected them when she was setting up my breakfast," mom replied. "They were really in the way. She just forgot to reconnect them."

I suppose it didn't hurt for them to be off for just a little bit. I thought about just reconnecting them but I wasn't quite sure how they went, or how the pump worked. This wasn't something I ever saw in the ER, and I didn't want to screw something up, so I would just wait for the nurse to come in.

"Is Rachel the nurse today?" I inquired. Mom shook her head.

"She's the CNA. I haven't seen a nurse yet."

That raised my eyebrows. It was 8:30 and a nurse hadn't been in yet? Then I remembered that they had six patients per nurse on this wing, and mom was probably one of their most stable ones. It wasn't like mom needed anything, and she had a call light if she did. I needed to relax and listen to Karen's advice to not nitpick the nurses.

Around nine, a young lady in pastel scrubs came in the room, walking hurriedly.

"Hi, Betty, sorry I'm so late," she said, breathlessly. "It is nuts out there today!"

Her nametag said 'Rachel, CNA', which I had already assumed, because she looked way too young to be a college graduate. She picked up mom's breakfast tray and asked if she needed anything else right now. Mom said 'no' and Rachel bustled back out the door.

After she left, I remembered I wanted to ask about the things on mom's legs. I didn't really want to ring the call light for something minor, since it sounded like they were pretty busy. I would just wait until the nurse came in for the morning assessment.

It was almost ten before a nurse came in. I could hear the constant activity in the hallway, so I knew they were busy. I didn't know if this was normal for them or if today was unusual, but there were a lot of people coming and going.

A short, plump woman wearing a nametag that said 'Lori RN' came into the room. Riley's extra had been all out front, but her extra was all out back. She sort of waddled when she walked and she didn't move too quickly. Her hair looked like it had been short and she was growing it out, but couldn't decide what to do with her bangs. They still fell forward on to her forehead, but they reached all the way to her chin.

She introduced herself in a flat voice as she walked directly to mom's chair. She set a small paper cup on the table that had pills in it, and briefly listened to mom with her stethoscope. She asked about pain and mom said she wasn't having any. Lori kept shaking her head side to side to get the hair out of her eyes, but it wasn't very effective. I really wanted to get a clip and pull her hair back for her. I'm not sure how she could see through all that.

Lori looked at mom's knee and I remembered that I wanted to ask about the SCDs.

"Are those supposed to be connected?" I asked, pointing at the sleeves.

"Yeah," Lori replied, slowly. She looked around for the tubing, but didn't move. I reached under the bed and grabbed the tubing I had seen there. She took it from my hand without a word and reached down to connect it. I watched surreptitiously to see how they connected, so I could just do it myself next time. She didn't walk over to the pump on the bed, so I assumed it was automatic and they just needed connected.

Lori gave mom her pill, which was the stool softener that I had guessed she was getting. Mom swallowed the pill and handed the cup back to Lori who tossed it toward the trash can. It missed the trash and landed on the floor. Lori just looked at it and then turned to walk out.

Ok, she wasn't the worst nurse I had ever met, but she wasn't the best either. I walked over and picked up the cup and put it in the trash can. She hadn't said anything about coming back, so I guess she was done with her morning assessment. I had noticed she didn't ask mom about pain, but maybe Rachel had already passed on that mom said she wasn't having any.

We sat there for about another hour, just chatting, and then mom decided she needed to get up to the bathroom. I rang the call light for the nurse, since mom still needed help with all her equipment. We sat there for several minutes waiting, but no one arrived. The morning hustle and bustle had died down a little, or at least it didn't sound as hectic out there. I peeked my head out the door to see if the light above the door was on, and it was. I could see a couple people standing at the desk at the end of the hall, all looking at pictures on someone's phone. None of them even looked in our direction.

I walked back in the room, silently fuming. I wasn't going to stomp out there and make a scene, but I wasn't happy that my mom couldn't get help. I could understand if they were all still running around, but if you have time to play on your phone, you aren't that busy. This was an argument I had with my co-worker, Jesse, all the time.

Finally, Lori came strolling in the room, looking bored.

"Yes?" she said, looking at mom.

"I need to go to the bathroom," mom told her. She was already starting to get situated on the edge of the chair, so it looked like she needed to get there soon.

"Oh, I'll go get Rachel," Lori said and walked back out. I stood there, flabbergasted. Why didn't she just help my mom? She was already here!

Mom was starting to look decidedly uncomfortable. I started getting everything ready in anticipation of Rachel's arrival. I disconnected the SCD tubing and moved the walker over in front of her. She was no longer connected to the IV, so we didn't have to worry about the pump. I had pretty much decided I could handle this on my own when Rachel walked in.

"Sorry about that," she said, quickly, hurrying to help mom get up. "I was in a room with another patient. I had to finish up in there."

Which was all the more reason that Lori should have helped my mom. Not only was the patient not getting help on time, the poor CNA was getting run ragged.

Mom got to the bathroom fairly easily. She was moving around pretty well, I thought. She used the bathroom and took a few minutes at the sink to brush her hair and teeth. Rachel was just getting her back to the bed when Lori walked back in.

“The guy in 128 puked all over,” Lori said flatly, to Rachel. “He needs washed up and his bed changed.” She turned to walk back out without even looking at mom.

“I need to finish with Betty,” Rachel said, sounding frustrated. Mom was sitting on the edge of the bed, but she wanted to lay down and rest for a bit before lunch.

Lori sighed impatiently. “I’ll finish this,” she said, sounding irritated. “You go get 128.”

Rachel did a good job of maintaining her composure but I could tell she was furious. Lori was dumping the more difficult task off on her, and behaving horribly in front of the patient. I made a mental note to mention Rachel to the manager and commend her hard work.

Rachel apologized to mom and hurried out of the room. Lori walked over by the bed and just stood there as mom managed to get herself situated in the bed. Once mom was under the covers, Lori turned to walk out. Mom’s bedside table had been moved away, so she couldn’t reach any of her stuff, and the call light was still on the chair, but Lori didn’t seem to care.

“Don’t these things on my legs need reconnected?” mom asked. Lori stopped and turned around slowly then sauntered back toward the bed.

“Oh yeah,” she said, not sounding the least bit concerned. She connected the tubing while I made a point of bringing the call light and table over to where mom could reach them. If Lori picked up on the hint that she wasn't doing all of her job, she didn't let on. She just walked back out of the room without another word.

"Thought that nice girl yesterday said those things were important," dad observed. I had heard Leah say that as well, but today nobody seemed that concerned. Leah said she needed them until she was up walking around. Technically, mom had walked a few feet, but I didn't think that was that much.

It was after eleven o'clock and mom was going to nap for an hour, so there was no point in dad and I hanging around. We decided to go get some groceries and lunch, and come back later this afternoon.

It was still dark and gray outside, but it wasn't snowing. We meandered through the small grocery store and I picked up the few things I had noticed they needed at the house. I also got some healthy snacks for myself, so I didn't end up eating all the candy sitting in mom's room.

I was starting to get hungry, so I asked dad what he wanted to do for lunch. He suggested we eat at La Cantina, a small Mexican restaurant there in town. I had eaten there before and the food was delicious. It also came in normal size portions, so I didn't end up eating way too much and feeling miserable afterward. I thought that sounded like a fantastic idea and we headed over there.

We walked in the door to be greeted by the smell of spicy peppers and warm tortillas. I felt warmer already. The entryway was lined with pictures of people who had successfully eaten the famously hot wings that were served here. We got a table in the back corner near the kitchen and opened our menus while the hostess went to get us water and tell the waiter we were here. The restaurant also had upstairs seating and my mom had always preferred to sit up there. Maybe her knee surgery would change that, stairs might be difficult for awhile.

"Roberto!" a man cried out. It was Juan, our waiter, and he loved to use the Spanish version of my dad's name. I thought it was funny, because my dad had rosy skin, blonde hair and green eyes, and didn't look the least bit Mexican. Dad thought it was funny because he really liked Juan, and that was how they male bonded, I guess.

Juan walked over to dad and shook his hand heartily. He looked at me for a moment and then said, "Betty, you look younger today!"

We all laughed at that. I do look like my mom, even though I got my dad's green eyes. Shelby got mom's blue eyes, but other than that, she didn't look much like the rest of us. Andrew looked like dad, green eyes and all.

"Spicy green chili for lunch today," Juan told us. "I made it myself."

Spicy green chili would be just the thing to warm me up, but I also really loved their chile rellenos. I was torn between the two, so Juan said he would bring me a cup of the chili and a half order of chile rellenos. That way I didn't have to choose.

"It will be *delicioso, bonita,*" Juan promised me. "We have a new cook and he is amazing!"

Then he gathered our menus, winked at me and added, “And he’s single.”

Sheesh.

Chapter Ten

We got back to the hospital a little after 8 o'clock the next morning. I hadn't managed to catch Dr. Lytle yesterday afternoon, but I didn't get too worked up about it. It was fine if mom didn't go home until today. I was hoping we would have discharge orders sometime this morning.

Mom was already sitting up in the chair, with a breakfast tray in front of her. I was glad to see her out of bed so early. Riley had been on last night, again, and he seemed to like to get his patients up and moving. I thought that was fantastic.

"Hi mom," I said, giving her a hug. "How did the night go?"

"Ok," she replied. "I slept pretty well, except for the beeping."

"What beeping?" I asked.

"Well, those things on my legs kept coming loose, and every time they did, the pump would beep. The noise kept waking me up."

"What happened when it beeped?" I asked. I didn't know much about these things.

"Riley would come in and readjust it and then it would work fine for a while," she replied.

"Did the cuffs squeezing bug you?" I asked. Leah had said some people really didn't like having the SCDs on.

"Well, I could feel it," mom replied. "I didn't feel yesterday when I was up in the chair."

Everything feels worse at night, especially if you're trying to sleep and can't. But part of the day, the cuffs weren't even attached to the pump, and I wondered if the pump wasn't working even when it was attached.

"How is the knee?" I changed the subject to one I hoped was positive.

"Good. A little tender this morning."

I tried to look at it, but it was still covered by a white stocking. Nothing looked too out of the ordinary through the Ted hose, though.

"That sock feels really tight, too," mom added. The left leg had been more swollen than the right from the beginning. Mom tried to reposition the leg and grimaced when she did it.

"When was your last pain pill, mom?" I asked.

"Right before I got out of bed," she replied.

"Did it not help?" I asked. It had only been two hours, she should still have some pain relief from that dose.

"A little," she hedged. "I don't know, it just hurts different today."

Uh-oh. That didn't sound good.

"What do you mean?" I asked. I could tell something was wrong, but she was always quick to brush off worries, at least when they were about her.

"It hurts farther down," she explained. "Yesterday, it was just in the knee, but now it's more down in the calf. And it feels, I don't know, achier. Is that even a word? It aches all of the time, instead of just hurting when I move."

I didn't have any experience with knee surgery, so I didn't know if that was cause for concern or just normal healing process. But the nurse who worked on the surgical unit and took care of knee surgery patients all the time would be able to shed some light on the subject.

As if on cue, Lori ambled through the door, holding the paper cup of mom's pills. She glanced at me and dad but didn't say anything to us.

"Here, Betty," she said, setting the pills on the table. Mom picked up the cup and dutifully took the pill inside it. From where I was standing, it looked like she was just getting the stool softener still.

I could tell my mom wasn't going to say anything to Lori about the leg hurting. Mom didn't like to complain, for one, but even if she wanted to say something, Lori's demeanor would stop her cold. So I decided to step in.

"Lori, mom said her leg is hurting worse today," I said, trying to keep my tone casual. "And she says it hurts farther down in to her calf. Is that normal?"

Lori shrugged and said, "I'm sure knee surgery hurts." I had a flashback to one of my dad's post-op nurses, who curtly dismissed dad's pain with 'well, it hurts to have surgery.' My blood started to heat up, but I tried to stay calm. Just because dad had a bad experience didn't mean mom would. Leah had said that they just started doing these procedures recently, so the nurses didn't have that much experience with them.

"I'm concerned that it hurts worse today than yesterday," I said, pointedly. "That doesn't seem like normal surgical pain."

A look of irritation flashed across Lori's face. I wasn't trying to nitpick her nursing, I just wanted to make sure that this was normal, because some sixth sense deep in my gut was telling me that it wasn't.

"Well, I've never seen a patient have that happen," she finally admitted. "But I don't know if it's really anything to worry about."

"What did Dr. Lytle say?" I asked mom. I assumed he had been through at the crack of dawn again.

"He hasn't been here," mom replied.

"He had a family emergency," Lori said. Mom gasped and Lori hastened to clarify, "His wife's car slid on some ice and ended up in the ditch. She's fine but he had to go get her out and take the kids to school. He'll be through later today."

I couldn't begrudge the doctor having a family emergency. At least I would get to talk to him when he came through on rounds today. I had been certain that we were going to get to take mom home later today, but I really wanted to make sure she was okay before we left.

Lori did a brief assessment of mom, and I tried to act like I was looking at the newspaper so she wouldn't feel scrutinized. Nobody likes to work under the microscope, and I knew firsthand how uncomfortable it was to try to do my job with people staring at me intently.

She seemed satisfied that nothing was too out of the ordinary, and turned to go. As she was walking out, Rachel came in with a stack of linens.

"Good morning, Betty," she said, brightly. "I'm here to give you a bath."

"Oh, that will feel good," mom sighed. "I feel sticky and itchy."

"Isn't funny how sweaty you can get just laying in bed?" Rachel asked, laughing.

I usually feel that families don't need to be an audience to the bath, mostly for the patient's privacy and dignity. However, I really wanted to see her leg without the stocking on it, just to be sure.

"Rachel, do you mind if I watch you take the Ted hose off?" I asked. "I'll leave after that. I just want to see the leg."

“No problem,” Rachel agreed easily. She had set the stack of linens in the bathroom, and knelt down by mom’s chair to pull off the stockings. She touched the left leg first, and mom winced a little.

“That leg hurts this morning,” mom explained.

“Ok, I’ll be careful,” Rachel promised. She carefully peeled back the stocking, and mom continued to grimace while she did it, but there was no way Rachel could have been any gentler. It was too soon for more pain meds, so she was stuck with toughing it out. Even though I knew there was no option, and that it would be over quickly, I still felt a stab to my heart at seeing my mom hurt.

The leg didn’t look so great once it was uncovered. The bandages were still in place, and the area of bruising inside the knee was still there, although it looked a little more colorful without the stocking over it. The whole leg, from ankle to mid-thigh, was red and swollen. There were ridges dented into the swollen tissue wherever a wrinkle in the stocking had been.

Rachel peeled off the stocking on the right leg and I compared the two legs. The left leg was significantly more swollen, but I think that was expected to some extent. But the fact that it was red and painful made me a little nervous.

Rachel had a funny look on her face, and I suspected she recognized that something wasn’t right. She had seen other patients after knee surgery, and the appearance of mom’s leg seemed to bother her.

“Did Lori see this?” she asked, politely restrained.

“Well, not without the stocking,” I replied. “We told her about it hurting more.”

“I think she should see this,” she said, trying to keep her tone neutral. I agreed and since I was starting to get antsy, I seized the opportunity to do something.

“Why don’t you get mom started in the shower, and I’ll go get Lori and have her come in there and look at it,” I offered.

“Oh, you don’t have to-“ Rachel started to protest but dad cut her off.

“It’s best to give her something to do when she starts to twitch like that,” he said, matter-of-factly.

Rachel tried to fight a smile but failed. I would have protested except it was completely true. Rachel agreed to start the shower while I went looking for Lori.

There were a couple people sitting at the nurses’ station, but none of them were Lori. I knew better than to go nosing in patient rooms looking for her, so I walked up to the desk. The clerk looked up at me and smiled.

“Can I help you?” she said, cheerily. She had blonde hair in a braid and a colorful headband that coordinated with her colorful scrubs. Maybe she was trying to channel the vibe of a tropical vacation.

“I’m looking for Lori,” I replied.

"She's in a room right now. Can someone else help you?" she asked.

"My mom is in room 134, Betty Sanford, and we were going to have her look at the leg while mom is up in the shower," I explained.

"Oh, ok. I'll let her know as soon as she comes out," the clerk offered helpfully.

I thanked her and walked back down to mom's room. That errand didn't use up nearly enough of my time and energy, but I couldn't think of anything else to do.

Dad looked up at me when I walked back in.

"She's busy, but she's going to come here when she's done," I told him. He nodded and went back to reading the paper.

Rachel had finished the shower and mom was dressed in a fresh gown. She brushed her teeth and combed her hair and then headed back to bed. Rachel had suggested that laying down and elevating the leg might help the swelling, and mom thought that sounded like a good idea.

Lori still hadn't come in, but Rachel said she would just leave the stocking off for now, so Lori could see the leg. Mom looked relieved to have the stocking off for awhile. Her swollen, tender leg didn't feel too good being squeezed into the tight elastic.

Mom looked pretty worn out, and she was grimacing with movement. It was almost 10 o'clock, so it was about time for the next dose of pain medication. We could ask Lori for it when she came in to check out the leg.

Lori didn't appear for another fifteen minutes, and she didn't seem too thrilled with being asked to come down here. She walked a few feet in to the room and then just stood there.

"Rachel said you want me to look at your leg," she said, bluntly. That wasn't exactly what Rachel had said, I was sure of it. Lori wasn't looking at mom's leg just to placate an overanxious patient. Lori needed to look at mom's leg because the patient, a nurse and a CNA all thought there was something wrong with it. I just bit my tongue. Lori would see in a minute why we were so concerned.

Lori raised the blanket off mom's left leg and stared at it for a minute. She looked like she wasn't sure what to make of it.

"Huh," she said, reaching down to touch the leg. Mom winced a little, and I interjected,

"She's having more pain, now."

Lori continued to look at the leg in bewilderment. "I've never seen one look like that," she finally admitted. She covered the leg up and stood there, uncertainly.

"Is Dr. Lytle on his way?" I asked, politely. "I think he would want to see that."

"He's coming in later," Lori repeated. I really wanted her to call Dr. Lytle and tell him about the leg, so he could decide if he needed to come sooner. That was sort of what the doctors expected of the nurses, to keep them up to date on changes in the patient's condition. Lori didn't seem too motivated to call him, though.

"He'll see it when he gets here," she said. She turned to walk out without even asking mom about pain.

"Can she have more pain medicine?" I called out as she was leaving. She stopped but didn't turn around.

"Yeah, I think so," she said, impatiently. "I'll get it in a minute."

I was liking Lori less and less. She was lazy and rude, and she didn't seem to care that something was wrong with my mom. Maybe something wasn't wrong with my mom and it was just normal swelling, but I really wanted to hear that from the expert.

Mom was looking pretty rough by now, and I hoped Lori hurried up with the pain pills. She must have picked up on my impatience, because she was back within a few minutes with some pills in a white paper cup.

"Here, Betty," she said, holding the cup out to my mom. Mom took the cup of pills, but she didn't have her water glass. It was sitting on the bedside table, which had been pushed out of the way when mom was getting back to bed. Lori just stood there, staring at her.

"Are you going to take them?" she asked, sharply, glaring at my mom.

"She needs water!" I snapped. I was about done with being polite to this horrible nurse. I grabbed the water glass and brought it over to mom. She swallowed the pills and started to hand the empty pill cup back to Lori, but she had already turned around and was walking away.

I set mom's water glass back on the table and moved it up next to the bed so she could reach it. I took the empty pill cup and put it in the trash. I noticed the blue cuff laying on the floor and I realized that mom didn't have the SCDs back on. She also didn't have the stocking back on the left leg.

I knew how to put them back on her, but she looked so miserable, I decided to wait until the pain pills had kicked in before I started moving her leg around. I paced around the room, picking stuff up and moving it around, trying to distract myself.

"Y'know," dad said, slowly, "Dr. Lytle gave us his cell phone number and told us to call him any time."

I stopped and stared at him. I knew what he was hinting at when he said that. Did I want to go over the head of our staff nurse and call the doctor directly? That was usually frowned on by hospital staff, and I didn't want to cause problems for my mom. But that was the same thought I had had when my dad was taking a turn for the worse, and it turned out that I really needed to cause problems because that was the only way to get him help.

My head, which usually overthinks things, said not to do it, but my gut said something was wrong and I needed to do something about it.

Dad must have seen the internal struggle and final decision in the expression on my face, because he just handed me a slip of paper. I looked down and saw it was the phone number of the doctor.

I grabbed my cell phone and dialed, before I talked myself out of it. A pleasant and familiar voice answered on the second ring, “Dr. Lytle here.”

“Dr. Lytle, this is Allie Sanford, Betty Sanford’s daughter,” I started out smoothly. Nurse mode kicked in, and I continued, “I’m sorry to bother you but mom’s leg is very swollen and painful and I am concerned about it. I wondered when you would be able to come in and look at it.”

I kept my tone cool and professional, just like I was calling a doctor from work. Dad raised his eyebrows, looking impressed.

“Oh no!” he said, sounding genuinely concerned. “That’s odd, no one has called me about it.”

“Well, Lori didn’t think it was of concern, but I can’t help feeling that it is,” I said, a note of urgency creeping into my voice. I didn’t want to sound alarmist, but I wanted to make him understand that this was serious.

“Ah, it’s Lori,” he said, knowingly. “Well, I’m glad you called me, Allie. I’ll be over there in ten minutes.”

"Thank you," I gushed gratefully. I was so glad that he was looking at my mom's leg right away that I didn't even care if Lori was mad at me.

"Oh, and I won't mention this call," he said, conspiratorially. He must have felt my anxiety about the nurse, and I was thankful that he knew how to handle the situation tactfully.

I disconnected, and glanced at dad, who was smiling slyly. I just smiled back.

Dr. Lytle arrived ten minutes later, just as promised. He stopped at the desk and hung his jacket over the back of a chair, as if he was just here for normal rounds, but instead of looking at charts first, he headed straight to mom's room.

"Hello, Betty" he said warmly, as he walked in. He glanced at us and added, "Good to see you, Bob. And thanks for calling me, Allie."

Doctors sometimes get a bad reputation for supposedly not wanting to be 'bothered' by nurses calling. But the good ones want nurses to call, they want to know everything that is going on with their patient. I was glad we had one of the good ones.

He walked over to the bed and pulled the covers off mom's leg. He scowled when he saw it, and gently reached down to feel around the knee.

"Wow, that's warm," he remarked, as he was feeling her leg. He checked the pulses on her foot and looked at the dressings on her knee.

"I agree, it doesn't look good," he said, after checking her over thoroughly. "It could be a couple of things. I'm going to order some blood tests that will help us figure it out."

He covered mom's leg with the blanket again. "I'm going to go look over your labs and vital signs, Betty," he said. "Then I'll stop back and chat with you."

"Does she need that stocking and cuff back on?" I asked. I knew mom didn't want tight things on her already tender leg, but I didn't want to have more problems than we already did.

"Let's wait on those for now," Dr. Lytle replied. "I'll be back in a bit."

Mom looked relieved at hearing that. I didn't want to cause my mom more pain, but I knew that sometimes the stuff that is good for us doesn't feel so good. But if Dr. Lytle didn't think she needed them right now, I was satisfied with that.

Mom was starting to look a little sleepy, now that the pain meds were working. I didn't want to wander off anywhere until I heard what else Dr. Lytle had to say. I perched in a chair and tried to relax, which looked about like a giraffe doing yoga- it just didn't look natural.

I decided to check my phone as a distraction, and saw four new text messages. Andrew and Shelby were both wondering how mom was doing, Lacey said that she hoped everything was going okay, and Jake wanted to know if I had punched anybody yet. I giggled a little at the last one. I tapped out responses to everyone inquiring about mom and sent them.

The medical field is pretty intense to work in sometimes, and there are some things that only another medical person can understand. Jake knew he didn't have to ask me how my mom was, because everyone else was already asking me, and besides- if she wasn't doing well, I would have told him already. But Jake knew that while everyone was bombarding me with questions and expecting me to handle any problems, no one was worried about how I was doing. It was nice to have someone care about how I was holding up. Jake really was a good friend to have.

I sent him a text telling him that mom's leg was swollen, but the doctor was here to look at it now, so no punches had been thrown.

'*Dang, I was excited to hear the story,*' he texted back. I smiled at that.

'*Stay tuned for updates,*' I texted back. I was pretty sure there would be no need for aggression, but it was fun to joke around with Jake. Something to laugh about was a welcome distraction right now.

Dr. Lytle was gone for quite a while, but he finally returned, apologizing as he came back in.

"Sorry, another guy was having problems, so I got pulled in there," he explained. He looked a little harried, so the other guy was probably not doing well. That would be the downside of having four patients in the hospital at one time- figuring out who needed you most.

"There's a couple things that might be going on," he started out, looking at me and dad. He glanced over at the bed but mom was now asleep, so he just spoke to us.

"It could be infection, which would cause the warmth, redness and swelling in the leg," he continued. "But her temperature and heart rate are normal, and they usually go up with infection. It could also be a blood clot in her leg, something called a DVT. That causes the pain and swelling too."

He paused for a moment and dad spoke up. "How does the blood clot get there?"

"Well, it is always a possible complication after surgery," Dr. Lytle explained. "We try to prevent it with the SCDs, which help keep the blood moving so it can't form a clot."

"Those were off for a good part of yesterday," I interjected. "They forgot to reconnect them, and even after they did, I don't think the pump was on."

Dr. Lytle mulled this over, looking none too pleased. "Well, we need to figure out which thing is going on, so we can treat it."

I nodded in agreement.

"I'm going to check some labs, which will give us our answer," he said. "I'll tell them to call me if any of the results are abnormal."

He glanced down at his watch and I did the same, noting with surprise that it was after noon. No one had brought a lunch tray in for mom, not that she was interested in eating.

"I'm going to see my other patients here and then head over to the clinic," Dr. Lytle said. "I've got patients pretty stacked up from my little adventure this morning. I'll write an order for the labs and to call me with results, and if the d-dimer is normal, they can put her SCDs back on."

I nodded, knowing the d-dimer would indicate whether or not she had a blood clot. If she did have a clot, we wouldn't want the cuff squeezing her leg and possibly breaking the clot loose.

"I'll be in touch," Dr. Lytle said, as he turned to leave. "But call me if you need to," he added emphatically.

Dr. Lytle walked out and I slumped back in the chair. Nothing to do now but wait.

"So, what happens if there's a blood clot?" dad asked me. I figured he hadn't asked the doctor any questions because he knew he could just ask me. I didn't mind this time around, because I knew what was going on.

"The blood test will tell us if there's a clot, and then they give her injections of a drug to prevent clotting," I told him. "That keeps the clot from growing and her body breaks down the clot that is there."

"Why don't they want that cuff back on?" he asked. "Isn't it going to help her if she has a blood clot?"

"It helps prevent the blood clot from forming," I replied, "but if she already has a clot, the cuff squeezing her leg could make the clot break loose. It goes through the heart and then to the lungs, which is pretty serious."

Dad just nodded quietly as he processed this information.

"Which of those two options is worse?" dad asked. I just shook my head, not sure how to answer.

"Neither one is great," I finally said. "But there's a treatment either way, so she's going to be fine."

Rachel stuck her head in the door and saw mom was sleeping soundly.

"I'm just going to send her lunch tray back, if that's okay," she said to me. "I don't think she feels like eating and she'd probably rather sleep. When she wakes up, we can get her something."

I nodded and Rachel headed down the hallway. It sounded like there was quite a bit of commotion down the hall, so they were all pretty busy. Maybe it was the room with Dr. Lytle's patient that was having problems.

I was getting hungry, but I didn't really want to leave mom right now. Dad read my mind again.

“Why don’t you go grab something from the kitchen downstairs,” he suggested. “I’ll stay with her until you get back and then I’ll go.”

I nodded. I knew it was silly to have one of us stay in the room all the time. It wasn’t like something major was going to happen in thirty minutes time, and she had a nurse watching over her. Well, technically she did. Lori wasn’t being too attentive. I couldn’t explain why I was nervous, so I was glad dad didn’t ask. I just grabbed my wallet and headed downstairs.

The cafeteria was serving roast turkey and dressing with gravy, which seemed perfect on this cold, wintery day. I could definitely use some comfort food right now. I snagged a piece of apple crisp as well, marveling at how well they disguised their fruit on the dessert counter.

I didn’t feel like sitting in the cafeteria by myself and eating, so I just took my tray back up to mom’s room. As soon as dad saw what they were serving, he hopped up and headed downstairs himself. Dad really liked turkey and stuffing.

I ate my food slowly, lost in thought. I had been so sure that this hospital trip would be different from the last one. Mom would have surgery, feel better, hop out of bed and go home. I had it all perfectly planned out in my head.

So why didn’t it work out that way? Was God trying to teach me something? I was certain I had learned all the hard lessons the last time. I didn’t feel like going through all this again. What was the lesson I had failed?

Oh, yeah- trust. I was supposed to trust God. That was easier to do when He was following along with the plan I had constructed. Why did things have to get complicated? And why did I have to keep learning the trust lesson through my parents getting sick? Couldn't I just get in a car accident or something? I didn't like watching my parents suffer, I would rather it be me. I was sure that would be easier.

I was sitting there, with my brow furrowed and my fork poised mid-air and not moving, when dad walked back in with his lunch. He looked at me and smiled.

"You arguing with God again, Allie-cat?" he said, laughing softly. I was nothing if not predictable. My dad seemed to have this unshakeable faith that kept him from ever worrying. Even when he was getting ready to go into open heart surgery, he was unflappable. He knew God would take care of him, and dad was actually the one who was reassuring me that he would be ok.

I told myself that dad had a lot more years to practice trusting God and that's why he was better at it. That pacified me a little, at least.

"I was just so sure this time would be different," I confessed. "We wouldn't have any problems and mom would just get better and go home."

"Well, that may still happen," dad reminded me. "This is just a little bump in the road. Like you said, there's a treatment for her, so it's going to be fine."

I had said that, hadn't I? I guess I needed to listen to my own advice. Mom was going to be fine, she was just going to spend a couple extra days in the hospital. I needed to trust God and just relax.

Like a giraffe doing yoga.

Chapter Eleven

I finally gave up on sitting and relaxing and decided to go for a jaunt around the hospital. I needed to move and nothing significant was going to happen in the next hour. They would draw her blood and then it would take a while to get results, so there was nothing to do but wait. I was almost as bad at waiting as I was at trusting.

I told dad I was going for a walk for a little bit. He nodded, without looking away from the TV. Some game was playing, which seemed to be a perpetual thing. I didn't know if people were playing sports around the clock, or if it was old footage.

I wandered around the hallways, trying not to look too suspicious. It seemed a little busier in here today. I would have thought, in this cold weather, people would want to stay home by the fire. Of course, most people in the hospital didn't come in just because they wanted to.

I walked past the waiting room we had sat in while mom was in surgery. I glanced in briefly as I passed the door, and I could see an older man sitting in the corner chair, with his head tipped back against the wall, sleeping. I could almost swear it was the same guy. I still marveled that anyone could sleep like that.

I found a secluded stairwell at the end of one hall, so I trotted up and down the single flight of stairs a few times. I needed to get some blood moving as well as burn off some nervous energy. I usually exercised a few times a week, so I was getting stiff and lazy, just sitting around. I was surprised at how quickly I got tired with that little bit of work. I needed to get out and move more. Too bad the hospital didn't have a workout room, like hotels did.

I meandered through the gift shop, browsing the racks of cards for funny ones. I liked to use humor to relieve my stress, and humor was on short supply today. Most of the cards were serious and thoughtful, but some were funny. Some were kind of dumb, and some were so dumb, they were funny.

I found a magazine to distract myself and bought it. I resisted the rack of sweet treats standing by the cashier, and I was pretty proud of that. I took my purchase and wandered back to mom's room, since I couldn't think of anything else to do.

Dad was still in the chair and mom was still asleep. It was almost 2 o'clock, and this day was starting to feel really long.

"Did they draw her blood?" I asked dad.

"Yeah, some gal came in and poked her," he replied. "Had a terrible time, too."

I glanced at my mom and saw the adhesive wrap on her elbow from where they had drawn blood. It was odd that they had a terrible time getting blood. Mom had great veins and usually even the beginners could get blood with no problem.

I settled in to the chair with my magazine, and started leafing through the pages of advertisements. I got to page 26 before there was any actual written content, and I was starting to feel like I had gotten tricked out of five dollars. And that I needed new shampoo and a wrinkle cream.

My phone buzzed with a text message. I opened it and saw it was from Jake, which made my worries about wrinkle cream vanish.

'*How is the weather there?*' he wanted to know.

'*Cold with a little snow. They're predicting a storm,*' I informed him.

'*Same here, so everyone flooded Wal-mart for supplies. And then someone pulled the fire alarm.*'

That didn't sound like a good day for the fire department. Evacuating public places was a major hassle, because no one wanted to leave. Especially if it meant giving up their place in line.

'*Just as a joke?*' I asked.

'*He said he thought it was a light to call an employee for help*' was the reply. I could imagine how well that went over with the crew. I just shook my head in amazement at how ridiculous some people could be.

'*In spite of the words FIRE ALARM on it, huh?*' I joked.

'*I don't think reading was his thing,*' Jake wrote.

'Does Wal-mart even have call lights to get help? I've never seen one.'

'I don't think so. But he did get attention from an employee,' Jake quipped. I laughed at that, which made dad look over at me curiously. Then he saw I was on my phone and just went back to his game.

Mom started waking up, so I stashed my phone and went to her bedside to see how she was feeling. She looked a little out of it, but she had been taking pretty regular doses of narcotics.

"Hey, mom, how are you feeling?" I asked.

She blinked a few times, trying to clear her head. "Ok, I guess," she finally answered.

"Want a drink?" I asked, as a suggestion, really. They had stopped her IV because she was drinking so well, but now that she was sleeping more, that wasn't the case.

She nodded and I handed her the water jug. She took a long drink and then set it back on the table and laid back with a sigh.

"How's the leg feel?" I asked.

"About the same," she answered. "It still aches, and it's worse when I move it. Even when I just move my foot."

That wasn't good news for her recovery. Joints needed to move so they could stay limber as they healed. If her leg hurt every time she moved it, she wasn't going to move it much. I couldn't blame her for not wanting to, either, but I hoped we had an answer soon so we could start fixing what was wrong.

I looked at my watch. It was 3:30, which meant it had been over 4 hours since her last pain pill. I tried to estimate in my head how long it would be before the lab result was done. I knew the lab they were checking could take up to an hour to process, and I doubt that Madison's little hospital had the most up-to-date equipment.

"Do you think you can get in the chair?" I asked mom. "Or do you need more pain pills first?"

"Pain pills," she answered quickly. That told me how much pain she was in, because she usually hesitated before admitting she needed something. That must be where I get my foolish pride from.

I pressed the button to call the nurse, checking my watch to track how long it took her to respond. After six minutes, I heard Lori's voice in the hallway. She had gotten almost to the door of mom's room, but had stopped to have a conversation with someone who was apparently quite a ways down the hall.

We could hear her talking loudly about their plans to go out for pizza this Friday, and then told a story about her dog chewing up her shoes. It was obviously a personal conversation, and it was irritating me for more than one reason. I didn't want to hear her stories, I didn't want to hear them at that decibel level, and I really wanted her to stop socializing and come help my mom.

She finally finished her chat and waddled the remaining few feet into mom's room. She walked over to the wall to cancel the call light without saying a word and then turned to mom to ask her what she needed.

"I'm having pain again," mom told her.

"You've taken a lot of pain pills," Lori scowled at her. "That's not a good idea after surgery."

I couldn't believe this lady was trying to tell my mom not to take pain pills, when her leg was swollen and red. This wasn't a typical surgical recovery, which was obvious from the fact that we were urgently checking for which complication she was having.

"She needs to get up in the chair, and she can't move if she's in a lot of pain," I said, tersely. "Once her leg is healing properly, she won't need as much medication."

Lori glanced at me with irritation, but finally relented and said, "Ok, I'll be back," as she walked out the door. I noticed she didn't say she would be *right* back and I was sure we would be waiting a little while for those pills.

I walked over to check out mom's leg, something I noticed the actual nurse didn't do. I remember a nurse early in my career emphatically teaching me that pain is a warning. It means something is wrong and never disregard it, always go looking for what is wrong. Apparently, Lori didn't get that lesson.

The leg looked worse than before, or at least it seemed like it to me. It was still swollen and elevating it didn't appear to have helped any. I gently touched the skin and it was very warm. I felt her forehead in an unofficial check for a fever, and it felt fine.

"What are they doing for my leg?" mom asked. She had been asleep when Dr. Lytle explained it to us.

"They are checking your blood to see if it's a blood clot or an infection," I told her. "Once they know that, they can start the appropriate treatment."

"When will they know that?" mom wanted to know.

"I would think it would be any minute now," I replied, glancing at my watch again. "It's been a while since they drew the blood."

Mom glanced down at her arm where the adhesive wrap was around her elbow and remarked, "That girl had a lot of trouble with that."

I reached up and pulled off the wrap, since it only needs to be on for thirty minutes. There was already a bruise forming in her elbow crease where they had stuck the needle. And mom's vein was still looking as hearty and healthy as ever, so I really did not understand how someone couldn't find it.

Mom was starting to shift around in the bed more, grimacing each time she tried to move the leg.

"Mom, wait until you get some pain medicine on board," I told her.

"I have to go to the bathroom," she confessed. That wasn't going to wait until she had pain medicine on board, especially since we didn't even know when the pills would actually get here.

I helped her get to the side of the bed, and she sat for a moment, getting her bearings and gathering her courage. Finally, she stood up, wobbling slightly as I stood there holding tightly to her arm to steady her. We moved slowly toward the bathroom, and while she didn't look great, moving didn't seem to be making the pain worse. She got to where she needed to be without any major problems. I stepped out of the bathroom to give her a little privacy, at least. Usually, I tried to keep that personal boundary in place and let the staff take care of the more personal stuff. But we weren't getting great care from the staff today, and I wasn't going to make my mom sit there for twenty minutes while we waited for someone to help her.

She was able to get from the toilet to the sink using the handicap rails, and after she washed her hands, we were ready to get in to the chair. Dad had relocated to one of the 'visitor' chairs, so mom could have the recliner. I grabbed a blanket and threw it down on the chair before she sat. The back side of a hospital gown doesn't cover things very well, and no one wants their skin directly on the vinyl chair.

Mom got seated and leaned back with a sigh. It was amazing how much energy it could take to do such a simple task. I was worried that she wouldn't want to drink water, so she wouldn't have to get up to the bathroom.

“It hurts worse when it’s down,” she said, pointing to her leg. I carefully raised the foot rest so her lower legs were elevated, and she nodded that that was better.

Lori finally wandered back in with some pills, and looked perturbed when she saw mom in the recliner.

“I thought you needed pain pills, first,” she said, sharply. Mom looked too wiped out to even reply, much less argue.

“She had to go to the bathroom, and she couldn’t wait, so she just had to tough it out,” I replied, tightly. I was sort of waiting for her to tell me I wasn’t allowed to get her up, that I needed to call for help. Lazy Lori, however, didn’t seem to care that a family member was doing her job. She handed mom the pills, and at least handed her the water glass as well.

“What did her lab results show?” I asked Lori. I was getting really anxious about my mom’s leg and I wanted a diagnosis so we could start a treatment.

“I haven’t seen any results,” she said, sounding bored. She must have picked up on my tension, though, because she said she would look when she got done with this. Once mom had swallowed the pills, Lori walked back out of the room.

I politely waited about ten minutes and then walked out to the desk. Lori should have had plenty of time to look up the labs, and I would save her the trouble of having to walk back to mom’s room to tell us what she found. I was just being considerate, right?

Lori was sitting at the desk, with her cell phone in hand, looking at something on the screen. She didn't look up when I walked up, just kept scrolling through her phone.

"Lori?" I spoke up, as politely as possible. "Did you find the labs?"

She actually continued scrolling through her phone for a couple more moments before she finally looked up at me, as if she wasn't sure who I was. Then she realized what she was supposed to be doing, and turned to the computer screen beside her. She clicked through some pages and I was very careful not to try to see what was on the screen. The chart wouldn't necessarily be my mom's, so it was a big no-no for me to see someone else's information.

Lori finished looking through the pages and turned to me. "There's nothing in there yet," she replied, looking unconcerned.

"It's been well over an hour since they drew her blood," I pointed out. "Results should be back by now."

I wanted her to call the lab and make sure they had processed the blood, but she wasn't picking up what I was putting down. She just shrugged and repeated that there was nothing in the computer.

I turned around and walked back to mom's room before I lost what was left of my cool and slapped the nurse. It wasn't a big deal to call the lab, we did it at my job all the time. The automated machines required a tech to go over and start and end the test, and sometimes they got busy and forgot to push whichever button produced a final result. You called and reminded them and then two minutes later, you had your result. Unfortunately, I couldn't call the lab here. I was going to wait a little longer and then call Dr. Lytle again if I had to.

I got back to the room and told my parents the results weren't done yet. Mom looked a little more relaxed with the pain pills starting to kick in. I was trying to think of what I could do to distract myself, when a lady walked in.

She was middle-aged with wire rim glasses and short, curly hair that was going gray. She was wearing a white lab coat and carrying a plastic caddy full of small glass tubes with colored tops.

"Hi, I'm Jean, from the lab," she introduced herself. "I'm sorry I couldn't get up here sooner."

"Oh, they already drew her blood," I told Jean. Jean shook her head grimly.

"She didn't get a specimen," she informed us. "I'm sorry for the extra stick, but I still need to get the blood."

I was still not understanding exactly what happened. "So, the first girl didn't actually draw any blood?" I asked.

"She told me she tried but the vein blew," Jean replied. "She's new, and still has trouble sometimes. We're the only two on, and ER had some stat blood draws that she also couldn't get, so I had to go do that first. I'm sorry."

I took a couple deep breaths, so I didn't blow up on Jean, the nice lady from lab who was finally going to draw my mom's blood. We had been sitting here for almost two hours, waiting for lab results from blood that hadn't even been drawn yet. Lori apparently didn't know it hadn't been drawn either, if she was looking for results.

Jean got set up and looked at mom's arm. "Well, look at these beautiful veins," she said, admiringly. Mom smiled at her.

Jean drew the blood in about ten seconds flat. She didn't have any trouble getting into the vein, and after she got the blood, she efficiently wrapped the adhesive gauze around mom's arm.

"This can come off in about thirty minutes," she explained to mom, gathering up her supplies. She apologized again for the delay and promised to run the blood right away.

"I wish she had come the first time," mom commented, still looking impressed with how smoothly Jean had accomplished her task. It sounded like Jean was getting the short end of the stick today. Her partner couldn't do any of the blood draws, so she was doing the work of two people. I had been there, and it wasn't much fun.

Rachel came bustling in and looked happy to see mom was up in the chair.

"Are you feeling a little better, Betty?" she asked, kindly.

"A little," mom replied, polite as ever.

"How about something to eat?" Rachel offered. They discussed the options and Rachel went off in pursuit of some soup and pudding. Mom hadn't eaten lunch, so I was glad she was hungry. At least she felt well enough to eat.

I had forgotten to ask Jean how long the test would take to run. I was watching the clock closely, just in case I needed to help Lori remember things. I was going to give it an hour before I went asking again.

Rachel returned with mom's late lunch, and she started to take a bite, but then stopped and looked at me.

"Did you get lunch?" she asked me. It never ceased to amaze me that her mom switch never turned off. Kind of like my nurse switch, I guess.

"Yeah, dad and I ate awhile ago," I assured her, and she started eat, relieved that her family wasn't going to starve to death. She made short work of the food Rachel had brought her, and I asked if she wanted anything else. She said she would wait until supper trays came, which wouldn't be too much longer.

I knew someone needed to go home and let Lady out, and I wasn't sure the cafeteria was even open for supper, but I didn't want to leave mom. Dad read my mind again, it seemed, and stood up, stretching.

"I'm gonna go let Lady out," he said to mom. "I'll come back in a bit and get Allison." My mom didn't like my nickname, Allie, so dad always tried to use my full name when he was around her. It sounded so stuffy and formal.

"I'll bring you back a sandwich," he said to me as he pulled on his coat. I wasn't sure exactly what he planned to bring, but I would eat anything, as long as I didn't have to leave mom. He hugged me and kissed mom good-bye and left.

"You sure do look nervous," mom observed. "Am I in trouble?"

"No," I replied, shaking my head. "It's just a little bump in the road. There's a treatment, whether it's an infection or a blood clot. I'm just impatient to find out which one it is so we can start the treatment."

"So, I don't need to get my affairs in order?" she joked, cocking one eyebrow at me. I laughed and finally relaxed a little. If she felt well enough to joke about dying, she obviously wasn't going to die. I needed to stop being such a worrywart.

We sat and chatted for twenty minutes and finally I decided it was time to check on lab results again. I walked out to the desk, where Lori was once again sitting, scrolling on her phone. Sometimes I wondered what people did to waste time at work before the Internet. Maybe they actually just worked the whole shift, but these days, it seemed like most people spent a third of their time playing on their phone. Which wouldn't bother me as much if it wasn't for the fact that they usually had work that needed done.

At least she looked up sooner this time, but when I asked about the lab results, she didn't even bother checking.

"They'll call me if it's abnormal," she informed me bluntly. I knew they were *supposed* to call, but poor Jean was getting run ragged down there and I wasn't sure she would have time to take care of that. Lori didn't seem concerned, though, so my hands were tied.

I was really glad that in less than two hours, we would have a new nurse. I really hoped Riley would be back tonight, because he would give my mother lots of attention and I could rest easy knowing nothing was going to slip by him. Like the SCDs being off, or the blood not being drawn for two hours.

I tried not to get to judgmental of Lori for missing a few things- we're all human and I've made my share of mistakes. I was just irritated that she acted like she was too busy to help mom, but then she was playing on her phone. I could understand a little better if she was actually busy.

I told mom there was no news yet, and she just nodded. She was leafing through the magazine I had bought earlier, and she seemed pretty comfortable. Maybe I really was overreacting.

Supper trays came and mom dug in to her chicken and rice, but not before she offered part of it to me. She also tried to give me her fruit cup and her dinner roll, as well as her carton of milk, but I assured her that she needed the nutrition more than me. She didn't try to offer me her dessert, which was a good thing, because it was a gooey brownie and I would have had a much tougher time turning that down.

Dad returned just before shift change at 7 p.m. with a grocery sack in hand. He had stopped at the grocery store and gotten food from the deli for us to eat for supper. True to his word, it was a sandwich, but it was turkey and Swiss on fluffy whole grain bread with tomatoes and honey mustard dressing. He had also brought apples and strawberries, and a container of broccoli salad. We sat and ate, listening to the bustle in the hallway as the night shift came on duty and got report on the patients.

Mom was starting to look a little peaked again, so I was relieved when Riley walked through the door shortly after report. He took one look at mom and his brow furrowed.

“Betty, darling, what did they do to you?” he cried out, dramatically. Mom smiled at him as best she could.

“Riley, it’s good to see you,” she said, sounding relieved. I guess I wasn’t the only one who was hoping for Riley back tonight.

“It’s been awhile since your last dose of pain med,” Riley said to mom. “Do you need more?”

Mom nodded and Riley told her he would be right back and walked out the door. He returned a few minutes later with her pills in hand. Mom took them gratefully and then Riley started checking out her leg.

"I can't believe how fast that happened!" he marveled. "It didn't look like that when I left this morning."

"We really didn't notice how bad it was until Rachel took her Ted hose off for the shower," I told Riley.

"She did say it was hurting a little, but I didn't think that was unusual," he said, "so I gave her some pain pills and that helped."

Riley seemed a little upset, as if maybe he had missed something and this was partly his fault. I knew that feeling, I had had it myself, but I didn't want him to beat himself up.

"It's ok," I assured him. "Once we know the lab results, we can get her back on the road to recovery."

"I called the lab," he told me, "but no one answered the phone, so they must be out doing a blood draw. There's not a result in the computer, so I'll keep calling them until I get an answer."

That was music to my ears. Riley was quickly becoming one of my favorite nurses. I always liked a nurse that went to bat for their patients.

I knew we were safe to go home now that mom was in good hands, but I still wanted to know what the lab results were. It wouldn't be much longer, I figured we could hang out for a little bit.

Mom's water pitcher was empty, so I decided to fill it while I waited. I had seen the little kitchenette in the hallway with the ice machine in it, so I grabbed the jug and headed down there. Riley was on a phone in the hallway at a small desk between rooms.

"There's nothing in the computer," I overheard him arguing with someone. There was a pause, and then he sighed, "All right, call me when it's done."

He hung up the phone and turned to see me standing there.

"They forgot to start the machine," he said, dejectedly. "It will be another twenty minutes. I'm really sorry."

"Hey, at least you called," I reassured him. "I'm grateful for that."

He smiled at what I didn't say, which was that Lori wouldn't even call. He promised to come tell us when he got the call.

I filled the pitcher with ice and water and walked back to the room. I updated mom and dad on the expected time for the lab result, adding that I wanted to stay until we got it and then we could head home. Dad just nodded, I'm sure he already knew that was what my plan was.

A knock came at the door, accompanied by a nasal-pitched voice asking, "Betty Sanford?"

I turned to see a sixty-plus woman standing at the door, carrying a vase of flowers and a box of candy. She had bottle-red hair curled and teased up all around her head, with blue eyeliner, bright red lips and a perfect circle of rouge on each cheek. She wore a crocheted red sweater vest stretched over her ample bosom with silk flowers and sequins affixed all over it. A small name tag identified her as Emmilynn and she was a hospital volunteer.

Mom looked at her and broke into a smile.

"Emmilynn! How nice to see you!"

Emmilynn bustled into the room, setting the goods on mom's bedside table, and then reached to hug mom. A cloud of perfume followed her into the room, and I tried not to sneeze.

"Oh, Betty, how are you? Are you okay? I was so worried, you havin' surgery and all, it's just a scary thing, and I was so worried about you, but how are you doing? Are you doing okay?" Emmilynn rambled on, words spilling over each other. She was touching mom's face and squeezing her hand and acting like mom was near death.

Mom tried to assure her that she was doing okay, but had trouble getting a word in edgewise as Emmilynn kept gushing about how worried she had been. I didn't bother to mention that mom had surgery two days ago, and this was the first we had heard of the very concerned Emmilynn.

She finally calmed down enough to tell mom that the flowers and candy were a delivery from a friend and handed mom the card. Mom opened the card and read it.

"It's from our neighbors," she said to dad. "That was sweet of them."

"Oh, isn't it wonderful to get flowers?" Emmilynn said, clutching her hand to her bosom. "It's just one of the best things ever. I just love to get flowers!"

It was a really beautiful bouquet of lilies, and I leaned over to inhale their scent.

"Of course, having surgery is no way to get flowers, it's just too painful," Emmilynn continued, turning toward me. "If you want to get flowers the easy way, you need to get yourself a boyfriend."

She looked at me pointedly and I looked back, bewildered. How did she know I didn't have a boyfriend? I glanced over at mom who just shrugged. Maybe Emmilynn was assuming I was single since I was here alone, but I didn't like this total stranger nosing into my personal life.

Emmilynn ranted on a little longer about how worried she had been and instructed mom to heal up fast and get home. Mom agreed that she would do her best, and Emmilynn hugged her a couple more times, then turned to leave. Just before she got to the door, she turned and pointed a long, red fingernail at me.

"When you find you a boyfriend, just remember this-" she admonished me, "if he doesn't bring you flowers, he's no good. But you find a man who brings you flowers, well, he's a keeper."

And she swept out the door with a flourish, leaving a trail of overwhelming floral scent in her wake.

Chapter Twelve

I was still a little stunned at getting dating advice from someone I didn't even know, when Riley came back in. He sniffed the air when he walked in and said,

"I see Emmilynn was here."

Apparently, her scent was her signature. Hospital workers weren't supposed to wear perfume, since it can cause breathing problems, but maybe volunteers didn't have those rules. Or maybe Emmilynn didn't follow the rules, which was the more likely explanation.

"Dr. Lytle is on his way in," Riley continued. "The d-dimer is really high, so it looks like it's a blood clot."

At those words, a chill ran over my entire body and the blood started to rush in my head. I had said I just wanted to know for sure what it was, but now that I knew for certain there was a blood clot sitting in my mom's vein, I was feeling a little panic-stricken.

I tried to keep it pulled together, though, because I knew dad was watching me to see how I reacted to the news. I nodded thoughtfully, waiting to see if Riley added anything. It seemed he was going to leave the rest of the explanation to the doctor, though. I would have done the same thing, because there were parts of the clotting cascade I didn't really understand and the doctor had a lot more years of school than I did.

"How's the pain, Betty?" he asked mom, looking genuinely concerned.

“Oh, it’s better,” she replied. “Still there, but not as bad.”

“Well, I expect Dr. Lytle here within fifteen minutes,” Riley told us. “I’ll be back in when he gets here.”

Ok, fifteen minutes to act cool, calm and collected, so mom and dad wouldn’t get worried. I could handle that.

Five minutes later, I was about to jump out of my skin. I had a terrible poker face and I’m sure mom and dad weren’t fooled that I wasn’t nervous. I thought about reading the magazine as a distraction, but it hadn’t even interested me that much when I was bored. I felt my phone buzz in my pocket and my heart sank. I wasn’t ready to answer any questions from Andrew or Shelby until we talked to the doctor.

I looked at it anyway, mostly out of habit, and it was a text message from Jake. Which was a welcome distraction right now.

‘*Weather says you’re getting a storm tonight*,’ it read. I hadn’t been outside all day, but any glimpses I caught through a window showed it was still gray and spitting snow.

‘*What day are you driving back?*’ his next message asked. It was nice to know Jake was worried about me being on the road in bad weather. Or maybe he just didn’t want to be on the crew that had to come peel me out of the car when I wrecked.

'*Not sure. Mom has a blood clot in her leg,*' I typed back.

'*Not good. What happens now?*' he wanted to know.

'*Waiting for the doc. We just found out,*' I replied. It was easier to talk about this with Jake. He wasn't going to bombard me with a hundred questions I didn't have the answer to.

'*Hold on,*' came the reply, which didn't make much sense. Hold on to what? My sanity? Although that was good advice, right about now.

About a minute later, my phone rang, and it was Jake calling. Oh, that was what 'hold on' meant. I answered on the second ring.

"Sorry, it's nuts here and I wanted to get to a quiet place to call you," he explained.

"What's going on?" I asked, curiously. Usually, the expression 'it's nuts here' wasn't conducive to personal phone calls.

"The guys are just wound up from all the calls today, and they're cooking supper, but it sounds like a locker room in there. So I'm back in the bunks now."

I nodded, even though Jake couldn't see me. I was getting so good at nodding silently, I looked like a bobble head doll.

"I missed something- I thought your mom was doing fine?" his statement came as a question.

"She started having pain and swelling in that leg this morning, and they finally checked her d-dimer and it's elevated," I told him. "The doctor is on his way in now."

"Didn't she have SCDs on?" Jake asked. I remembered that his dad had had hip surgery, so he had probably seen the blue sleeves on him as well.

"They were disconnected part of the first day," I sighed. "And even when they were connected, I don't think the pump was on."

"Dad's nurse was a Nazi about those things," Jake said. "Now I know why. How have the nurses been?"

That was a loaded question. I hesitated for a moment, not wanting to just blast all the nurses in my frustration. Really, we had only had one bad nurse, the rest were great.

"Ok," I hedged. "Riley is on tonight, and has been all three nights. He's really good. Our day shift nurse the last two days wasn't so great. In fact, I had to go over her head and call the doctor myself just to get him to come look at the leg."

Jake chuckled at that. "And how did that go over?" he wanted to know.

"Dr. Lytle didn't tell her I had called, he just conveniently showed up ten minutes later," I told him. "I get the feeling he knows what kind of nurse she is."

"So you didn't get in a punching match with the nurse, huh?" Jake teased me. "Allie, you're getting soft!"

I just laughed. Jake liked to tease me about being a scrapper, even though the only fights I had ever been in were with my siblings.

Just then, Dr. Lytle walked in the room and I sat up straight.

"Jake, the doc's here, I gotta go," I rattled off.

"Ok, I'll call you later," he said and disconnected. Mom's eyebrows raised slightly when she heard me say Jake's name, but mostly we were focused on Dr. Lytle and what he had to tell us.

He shrugged off his jacket and pulled a chair up by mom's bed to sit.

"It looks like a blood clot," he started out. "The d-dimer is high, which tells us you have clot somewhere in your body. It's nonspecific to location, although the obvious suspect is your leg. The definitive test is an ultrasound of the leg, but the ultrasound tech has gone home for the night and she lives twenty miles out of town, so in this weather, I hate to make her drive back in tonight. It wouldn't change my decision on what to do for treatment, so we can wait and get the ultrasound tomorrow."

He paused for a breath and looked around to see that all of us were still following along.

"The treatment is injections of low-molecular weight heparin," he continued. "You get the injections twice a day, and they keep your blood cells 'slippery' so they won't form more clots. Then your body breaks down the clot that is there, and once the vein is cleared out, all is well."

Mom mulled this over in silence and dad didn't seem inclined to ask anything either. None of us needed to ask how it happened, we had a pretty good idea what had brought this about. I jumped to the next most obvious question.

"How long does she have to stay in the hospital, then?" I asked Dr. Lytle.

"The good news," he laughed humorlessly when he said it, " is that she can give herself the injections at home, so once we know the clot is stable and she is able to get around without too much pain, she can go home. The amount of time it takes for the clot to completely clear depends on how big it was to start with, and everybody's system processes stuff at a different rate."

Mom seemed nonplussed at the mention of giving herself injections, but dad's eyes grew wide. Good thing Dr. Lytle didn't suggest a family member could give the injections.

"I'm really sorry this happened, Betty," Dr. Lytle apologized earnestly. "I know we tell patients that it's a possibility, but it's usually just a formality. I won't lie, the SCDs being off could have led to this. And some people are just more prone to make clots than others, and we don't find it out until something like this happens."

"Well, it's not the worst thing that could happen," mom said calmly. "It's certainly not your fault. I'm sure everything will be fine in the end."

Mom was right, everything would be fine in the end. This was just a minor setback and no reason to get all upset. A minor adjustment to the plan for recovery was all that was needed. She was such a practical gal.

"We'll give the first injection right away," Dr. Lytle continued. "I'll go write the order right now. I called Dr. Steitler earlier, so he knows what's going on too. I'll let you know if anything changes, and please"- he glanced at me meaningfully, "call me if you have any concerns."

He headed out the door, leaving us sitting in silence as we processed all the information. After a moment, I remembered my siblings and jumped up.

"I'm going to call Shelby," I told my parents. "Mom, do you want to call Andrew and Nicole? You can talk to the girls and then I can tell Andrew what's going on."

I had an ulterior motive there. It did accomplish two phone calls in the time of one, but I also knew that if Andrew heard mom's voice first and she sounded like she was okay, he wouldn't get as spooked when I had to tell him about the blood clot in her leg.

Mom's face lit up at the prospect of talking to her grandkids and she reached for her phone readily. I grabbed my phone and called Shelby, stepping into the bathroom so mom and I weren't trying to talk over the top of each other.

"Hey, 'Lis," Shelby answered on the third ring. The original plan had Shelby coming to Madison tomorrow and me going home, but that plan also included mom being at home by now. I had texted her earlier to let her know that things weren't going quite to plan.

"It's a blood clot," I blurted out, skipping right past 'hello'. "She has to stay in the hospital for a few days, probably."

"Is she going to be ok?" Shelby cried out.

"Well, it's serious, but not *that* serious," I assured her. "It's just a complication of her surgery, but she has to start getting injections to treat it. They don't know for sure when she'll get to go home."

"Well, I assume you are staying," Shelby commented drily. "Mother Nature isn't helping our plan any, there's supposed to be a wicked winter storm coming in tonight."

The road from Madison to Brighton wasn't terrible, but with snow this thick, the visibility was minimal and the plows had trouble keeping up. There was no point in Shelby risking her neck to get here when I was staying anyway.

Originally, I was going to go home when Shelby came over, but I had taken the whole week off work, thinking it would be a good mini-vacation for me. It was a good thing I did, because now I wasn't coming back when I had planned.

"Well, I guess we'll all stay where we're at and settle in for a snowstorm," I sighed. Blizzards were so much fun when I was a little kid. We got to miss school, and build a blanket fort in the living room and drink hot chocolate, watching out the window as the drifts piled higher. It had been a long time since I was excited about a snowstorm.

I got off the phone with Shelby and went back into the room to talk to Andrew. Mom was laughing, still on the phone, so the girls were obviously entertaining their Nana. Mom was such a wonderful grandma, I felt a little guilty that she didn't have grandkids closer to home. Then I reminded myself that it wasn't like I was deliberately withholding grandkids from her, I just hadn't met the right guy yet.

Mom finished talking to Cassie and Sammie and then chatted with Andrew briefly. I heard her say, "I'll let you talk to Allie," and then she handed me the phone.

"Hey, bro," I said, cheerfully.

"It's you," he said emphatically. "I've decided it's you. You're the magnet. Every time you're around, mom or dad ends up with something wrong."

I could hear the laughter in his voice, so I knew he wasn't serious. Anyways, he was right- every time something went wrong with their health, I was there.

I explained what Dr. Lytle had told us, and Andrew didn't have any other questions. I told him I was staying here and we were about to get snowed in.

After I finished talking to Andrew, I hung up and handed mom her phone.

"You're staying, Allison?" mom asked me, with a note of concern. "Don't you need to go back to work?"

"No, I took the whole week off," I told her. "The weather is turning bad, so it doesn't make sense for Shelby to try to drive here and me drive home."

Mom agreed that it made more sense for me to stay, especially with the weather getting worse.

"But why did you take the whole week off?" she wanted to know. She was looking at me intently, as if she thought I had known ahead of time that something would go wrong.

"I have a bunch of extra vacation time, and we've been short-staffed so I haven't been able to take any days off. Since my mom was having surgery, they couldn't deny my request, so I went ahead and took a whole week just to have a little extra time off," I confessed. At the time, I was just looking forward to a few days with nothing to do but watch movies and catch up on sleep. I hadn't actually *told* my boss I was staying the whole week with my mom, I just let her jump to that conclusion on her own. Of course, now I was actually going to spend the whole week with my mom.

"Well, I guess it's a good thing, since you're about to get snowed in here," mom admitted.

Riley came walking in with a small plastic syringe in his hand.

"I've got your first dose, here, Betty," he said to mom. "It needs to go in the abdomen."

He carefully repositioned her gown so her belly was partially exposed but the rest of her stayed covered. He gave the injection and then covered her back up.

"That wasn't too bad," mom said. "I'm sure I can do that."

Dad was staring intently at the TV, even though it was on a commercial for cat litter. He seemed quite determined to not see the injection being given. I found that amusing, because he had been fine with all of this when he was the patient.

Now that mom had her injection and everyone was updated, dad and I could head home. I had briefly considered sleeping in her room overnight, but I couldn't justify why I needed to stay, and I knew it would be a really bad night's sleep. I felt safe with Riley on watch. I gave him my cell number as well as the house phone number and he promised to call if anything happened.

We said good-bye to mom and bundled up against the cold. The flakes were getting bigger and coming down faster, and there was already four inches collected on the ground and piled on the cars. I helped dad brush the snow off the truck, while it warmed up. He had exchanged the car for the 4-wheel drive truck when he went home for supper.

It was beautiful and eerily quiet, with the snowflakes falling through the glow from the parking lot lights. It was weird how snow falling made it feel quieter, as if the flakes absorbed sound.

We drove home slowly on roads that were mostly unplowed. There were only a few other vehicles out, most people were home for the night. Now that we were headed home, I was incredibly exhausted.

There was a natural hot springs in Madison, and the thought of sinking into the steaming pool at the state bath house was very tempting. I usually packed a swimsuit whenever I came to visit them, just in case. However, this trip wasn't the usual visit, so I wasn't prepared. Besides, I would probably fall asleep and drown. I gazed wistfully at the pillars of steam rising from the pool as we drove to the house.

We got to the house and I headed straight for bed. I put my phone on the charger right next to the bed and made sure the ringer was on high. I crawled under the covers and was asleep before my head hit the pillow.

I woke up with a start, and had a moment of panic when I didn't recognize my bedroom. Then I remembered I was at my parents, and that I really had to pee. I got up and went to the bathroom, and then crawled back into bed.

I reached over and picked up my phone, just to check. I was sure I hadn't missed any calls, but I just wanted to make sure.

I was holding the phone in my hand when it loudly rang, and I jumped six feet in the air. It was a good thing I had just gone to the bathroom, or I would have wet my pants.

"Hello?" I answered breathlessly. I didn't recognize the phone number, and that wasn't a good sign.

"Allie, it's Riley," I heard. My heart was already racing, and my mouth went dry.

"Yes?" I croaked.

"Betty's having some trouble breathing," he said quickly. "Dr. Lytle is on his way. It could be a PE."

He paused for a moment, and I broke in, "We'll be right there."

"Ok. Drive safe," he said and hung up. I knew that Riley had more important things to do right then than talk to me on the phone.

Lady had been sitting in the doorway watching me, and as soon as I hung up, she barked loudly and then ran down the hall towards my parents' room, still barking.

Lady almost never barked, so she must have known something was going on. I pulled on my robe and headed down the hall behind her.

Dad was sitting at the edge of the bed, already pulling on a shirt.

"Heard Lady barking, so I figured something was up," he said.

"Mom's having trouble breathing," I said, a little breathless myself.

"I'll go start the truck," was all dad had to say. I scurried back down to my room and threw on clothes. I felt like I had just run a mile, I was breathing hard and my heart was pounding. I grabbed my cell phone and headed for the front door.

Lady was sitting there, looking worried. I stopped to pet her for a second, and thank her for being my lookout dog. Then I grabbed my coat and gloves and headed out the door. Dad had the truck started and was sweeping off all the snow that had accumulated in the few hours since we got home.

The outside world was buried in snow. I could barely make out the trace of the tire tracks we made when we came home last night. This was our first big snowstorm of the year, and usually I'm excited to see all that powder, but right now, I really would have preferred clear weather. I was thankful we had 4-wheel drive, because the plows in this sleepy little town were not keeping up with the snowfall.

Dad drove slowly down the street, following the few tire tracks that were there. Most people were staying home, dry and warm. We got to the hospital, where at least the parking lot was plowed. I could see the pickup with the blade on it driving back and forth, fighting a losing battle against the weather. The maintenance man was going to have a long night and day tomorrow. I had seen our crew work 36 hours straight, taking turns napping on a cot set up in their break room.

We got in the front door, brushed off the snow that was collecting on our head and shoulders, and headed quickly down the empty hall to mom's room. The dead quiet gave way to urgent voices as we got closer to the room. There were two nurses, a respiratory therapist, and Dr. Lytle crammed in that little room. We slid in along the wall, watching the scene fearfully.

Mom was sitting upright in the bed, with an oxygen mask over her face. Her breaths were rapid and shallow, and her neck muscles were straining with each breath. She looked frightened and exhausted at the same time, and my gut clenched at the sight. The respiratory therapist was listening to her back with a stethoscope, his eyebrows drawn together in concern.

"I just don't hear anything in this one lobe," he said, straightening and turning to the room. His eyes landed on us and his eyebrows raised. No one had heard us come in with all the bustle.

Dr. Lytle turned and saw us there and walked the few steps to where we were standing.

"It looks like she has a pulmonary embolism," he said, looking mostly at me. He looked a little frightened himself, and it was a good possibility he had never experienced this before either.

"We got an x-ray of her chest, which of course, isn't a conclusive test, but it's all we have right now," he continued. "She was getting out of bed to go to the bathroom and she suddenly began having respiratory distress. Her sats dropped, and you can see how she's breathing. We are planning to move her to the ICU."

"You have an ICU?" I blurted out, incredulously, before I could stop myself.

Dr. Lytle smiled wryly. "Of sorts," he said. "It's not open right now so we're waiting for a nurse to get here from home."

He glanced back at mom and ran a hand over his head and down his neck. He looked worried and a little overwhelmed.

"This is really more than we would normally handle here in Madison," he confessed to me, nervously. "I always transfer these patients out to Springfield. But with the weather like it is, no one is flying and they are closing the road, so we can't even send her by ground ambulance."

He was staring at mom distractedly while he talked. He paused for a long moment, lost in his thoughts, then took a deep breath and stood up straight.

"We're going to do everything we can," he said, firmly, turning back toward us. "I can promise you that. We'll get her through this."

I just nodded silently again, at a loss for what to say. It was nerve-wracking to know that they didn't really have the staff or equipment they needed to best help my mom, but there was nothing that could be done about it. Might as well make the best of a bad situation.

Dad and I stood there, silently, watching everyone hovering around mom. She was still struggling to breathe, and she had looked over at us and smiled briefly, but I knew we didn't need to get closer right now. The staff didn't need us in their way.

"Ellen Mayers had one of these," dad remarked, quietly. "That's what did her in."

Ellen Mayers was a lady in their church, who had been hospitalized for a minor procedure on her kidney and ended up never coming home. They hadn't even diagnosed the blood clot yet, when she just collapsed. They didn't find out what had caused her sudden death until they did the autopsy, and her death had hit the church hard. She was a much-loved woman.

"Well, if it's any consolation, dad, if the clot is going to kill someone, it usually does it right away."

He looked at me sideways for a moment. That tidbit of information was, ironically, our good news for the moment. The severity of the PE depends on the size of the clot that breaks loose- the larger the clot, the larger the area of the lung that gets taken down.

Riley came in and talked to the respiratory therapist. They determined that mom was stable for now and we were just waiting for the word to transfer her to the ICU. Mom was still working to breathe, but it didn't look quite as bad as it had. The staff were clearing out so dad and I moved up closer to the bed, reaching out to hold mom's hand. She looked frightened still, but relieved to see us.

I didn't want her to try to talk while she was having so much trouble breathing, so I didn't say anything to her. She grabbed my hand and squeezed tight, and I wasn't sure I would have been able to talk anyway. I blinked back tears, fighting to stay calm for my mom.

We had sat there in tense silence for about two minutes when my dad took mom's hand in one hand and my free hand in the other, and bowed his head.

"Lord, we need a little help here," he said, earnestly. "Betty's having trouble and I know You can help her. She needs You right now, Lord, so please help her get through this."

His voice broke slightly on the last word, and I held my breath to keep from crying. Dad had always seemed so strong in the face of adversity, and his faith was unwavering. Even when his own life was in jeopardy, he calmly trusted God to take care of him. I had always admired his ability to trust God when things weren't going so well.

But now my dad was even choking up at the possibility of my mom not making it through, and my heart clenched painfully. Emotion welled up in me and suddenly words were tumbling from my mouth.

"God, please help my mom, please, I need her and I need to have her just get better, and please, God, please-" I took a deep, shaking breath and continued, "please heal her. Amen."

"Amen," I heard my mom say softly, under her oxygen mask. I looked up at her, my eyes brimming with unshed tears, and she smiled softly and reached out to touch my face. I sat there, motionless, too overwhelmed to even talk.

Riley came striding in, breaking the silence, to announce that the ICU nurse was ready. He and another person were going to just transport mom in the bed down the hallway. Dad and I hastily stood up and moved to the corner of the room, while they got everything ready. There was a green oxygen tank laying on the bed and they connected her oxygen mask tubing to it. They stacked her other belongings on the bed around her and Riley tucked a chart under the mattress. He unlocked the brake on the bed and they started moving the bed out the door and down the hall.

Dad and I followed along behind them, not saying anything. The rest of the unit was peacefully sleeping, with all the hall lights turned down low, and I didn't want to make any noise.

The ICU was at the far end of the hallway, through a set of double doors. As we walked in, I was struck by how small it was. Bright fluorescent lights flooded the desk and rooms with a harsh glow. The nurses desk was almost bare, just one phone and computer sat there. The room they wheeled mom into was right next to the desk and had a large glass door, so the nurse could see mom all the time. The cardiac monitor above the bed was turned on with flat green lines running across it, since it wasn't connected to mom yet.

A middle-aged woman with short brown hair stood in the room and as they maneuvered mom's bed into position, she introduced herself.

"I'm Gina, and I'll be your nurse," she said to mom. She immediately began placing wires on mom, measuring her heart rate, blood pressure and oxygen level. Out of habit, I looked at the screen to see what her vital signs were, and I was relieved to see that her oxygen level was 95%.

Dad and I stayed out in the hallway, while Gina got mom situated in her room. She listened to her heart and lungs and checked out her legs, noticing the swelling in the left leg. She explained the routine to mom, how the blood pressure cuff ran automatically and her heart rate and oxygen were continuously monitored. She wasn't super cheery, but she was efficient and polite. Besides, we had just woke her up in a blizzard to come to work. I wouldn't be super cheery either.

She completed her very thorough assessment and then gave mom the call light, telling her to press it if she needed anything or had any new symptoms. Mom nodded and Gina walked back out of the room.

"You can go in now," she told us. "Thank you for waiting."

We walked in to the room, which looked and felt like a smaller, older version of dad's room in the ICU in Springfield. I hadn't really enjoyed our experience in the Springfield ICU and I had no desire to revisit it. Unfortunately, it looked like we were going to wander down that same path.

And I was about to get a serious lesson on trusting God.

Chapter Thirteen

Dad didn't head for the recliner like I thought he would. Instead, he pulled up one of the other chairs and sat next to mom's bed, holding her hand. It was a picture so sweet, I thought I might cry. They were such an adorable couple sometimes.

I pulled out my phone, dreading making these phone calls. It's really hard to convince someone their mom is okay when you just woke them up at 4 a.m. Everything feels worse in the wee hours of the night. I called Shelby first.

She didn't answer until the fourth ring, and then I got a mumbled something that sounded less like 'hello' and more like 'what'. Shelby was a sound sleeper and she didn't wake up well or quickly.

"Shelby, wake up, I need to talk to you," I said, trying to keep my voice quiet. I hadn't noticed any signs about not using my cell phone, but it was still rude to talk loud in the hospital. Or anywhere, really.

There was a long pause, and I thought she might have fallen back asleep when she finally heaved a sigh and said, "Ok, I'm awake. What's wrong?"

"The blood clot went to her lung," I said. "She's having trouble breathing, and they've moved her to the ICU."

"What?" she cried, sounding much more awake now. "That sucks! How bad is it?"

Being in the ICU can cover a wide range of medical problems, some more serious than others. We had seen our dad in the ICU, unconscious with tubes and wires everywhere, then in the ICU sitting up and talking to us, and then again semi-conscious and seriously ill. Since Shelby couldn't see mom, her imagination was probably running away with her and she was picturing the worst possible scenario.

"She'll be fine," I assured her. "She's on an oxygen mask, and she's working a little bit to breath, but her oxygen level is 95% so she's getting enough oxygen."

"So what do they do now?" Shelby wanted to know.

"Well, usually they would transfer her to Springfield, according to Dr. Lytle. But the road is closed, so that's not an option."

There was a long pause while Shelby pondered this. "What if she gets worse again?" she asked. "Then what?"

"Honestly, that's not likely to happen," I replied, hoping to convince myself as well as Shelby. "The worst thing that can happen, the clot traveling to her lung, has already happened, and it wasn't a big enough clot to take her out. Now we just wait for her body to break down the clot and we give her oxygen and whatever else she needs."

"Man, I don't want to go through this again," Shelby sighed. I totally understood how she felt, but I was trying really hard to keep a positive outlook.

"Hey, we got a happy ending the last time," I reminded her. "And we have an awesome doctor and a good nurse. It's all good."

Shelby was slightly pacified with that. Since I still had to call Andrew, I cut it short, telling her to call me when she woke up later. I was pretty sure I wouldn't be getting any more sleep tonight.

I dialed Andrew next, who answered on the second ring and already sounded wide awake. I told him about mom's change in condition and that she couldn't transfer out due to the weather. He didn't have any other questions, which was good, because I didn't have much for answers.

"I was just kidding earlier," he said earnestly. "I'm glad you're there with her."

"I know," I replied. "I'm glad I'm here too. I'll call you with any more news."

I hung up and stood there, uncertain of what to do next. If I could sleep like Shelby, I would just curl up in the recliner and conk out. Unfortunately, I couldn't sleep like Shelby, so my day was going to be long and exhausting. There wasn't really anything to do here, besides stare at mom and worry about how she was doing, and I don't think she appreciated being stared at nonstop.

Mom's few personal belongings had been shoved in plastic sacks and were sitting on the counter by the sink, so I took them out and put them away. As I was putting her cell phone and charger in the drawer on the night stand, I saw a Bible in the drawer and pulled it out. A sticker on the front said it had been placed there by the Gideons.

I sat in the recliner and kicked it back, opening the Bible to a page that had been bookmarked. It was the passage in Matthew that I had been trying to remember while mom was in surgery. I read through chapter 6, the familiar words comforting me. I got to verse 27, one I had repeated to myself often, "*Can any one of you by worrying add a single hour to your life?*" I closed my eyes and silently recited from memory the following verse, "*Consider the lilies of the field, they do not toil or spin.*" I felt a calming sense of peace steal over me as I laid there, remembering those words.

A beeping noise startled me, and I sat up abruptly, looking around. Mom was getting up to a commode beside the bed, and the beeping noise was her cardiac monitor, which had gotten disconnected. Gina was helping her with the transfer and dad wasn't in the room. I must have fallen asleep, because it was now almost 7 o'clock in the morning.

Mom saw me sit up and looked over at me with a smile. "Well, good morning, sunshine," she said. That was how she had always greeted me each morning when I came out of my room, and it always brought back happy childhood memories. Mostly of the breakfast she was cooking for me when she said it.

"Hi mom," I said. "Are you okay?"

"Yes, just needed a bathroom break and they don't want me to try to walk since I'm still having trouble breathing," she replied as she moved over to the commode. I didn't want to invade her privacy by being in the room while she was using the commode, but if I left right now, I was just going to expose her to the hallway when I opened the privacy curtain. Mom didn't seem to mind, so I stayed where I was.

I stretched and yawned, amazed that I had been able to fall asleep and stay conked out for two hours. I was glad for it, though, I felt a lot better now. I looked at my phone, out of habit, and there was nothing new on it. Which wasn't surprising, not many people are up texting and Facebooking at 5 a.m.

Gina assisted mom back to bed, and reconnected the monitor. Mom was still having trouble breathing, and it was a lot worse when she tried to move around. That would make sense, since she was basically missing a part of her lung. I wondered how long it would take before blood flow started getting past the clot again.

"We're going to change shift at 7," Gina told us. "I'll be in with the day nurse to see you before I leave."

"Where's dad?" I asked mom, after Gina had left.

"You were sleeping in the recliner, so Gina told him he could use the waiting room to lay down for awhile," mom explained. "He's just down the hall, she said. But there's no point in waking him up, nothing is going on. We might as well let him get some rest."

I agreed, and I'm sure dad would have too. Sitting around in a hospital room was really boring, and I wasn't too excited about a couple more days of it. I knew I didn't need to be there all the time, but it felt weird not to be. Besides, there wasn't much else I could be doing, especially in this weather. I needed to find a book to read, that would make the time go by a little faster.

I stood up and stretched again, and decided coffee was definitely a good idea. I told mom was I was going for a cup and I would be right back.

Gina was sitting at the desk, looking tired, with mom's chart in front of her. She must have been done with her charting, because she was just sitting there, resting her head on her hand and looking like she really wanted to go to sleep.

I stopped by the desk to visit with her, mostly out of curiosity.

"I didn't realize Madison had an ICU," I said, trying to sound nonchalant.

Gina smiled at that, with a knowing look on her face. "Well, it's almost never open," she said. "And if it is, it's usually some 90-year-old on a low dose nitro drip or something else pretty simple. Most of the shifts I'm on call for, I never get called."

"So, you're just on call for ICU?" I asked.

“Well, I fill in wherever they need me,” she said. “I don’t work full-time. We moved here from Omaha a few years ago and I was an ICU nurse there, so I fill in here.” She sort of laughed and added, “I don’t really keep my skills up, but usually I don’t need them.”

I’m sure the ICU in Madison was a far cry from the one in Omaha. We had a six-bed ICU in Brighton, but it usually only had a couple patients. I wasn’t sure what type of patients they took, but I did know that all our cardiac patients had to get flighted to Springfield.

“Well, I’m glad you were here last night,” I told her. She had seemed very competent and thorough when she took care of my mom. The nursing skills might be a little rusty, but they were still there.

Gina thanked me and I headed off to the cafeteria. I looked around as I was walking down the hall, until I saw a door labeled ‘ICU Waiting Room’. I peeked my head in to see if my dad was ok. The room had a couch, one chair, and one end table. It was even smaller than the surgery waiting room had been. Dad was stretched out on the couch with a pillow and blanket, so I left him alone.

I got to the cafeteria and headed straight to the coffee pot. Now that I could smell food, though, I realized I was hungry. I wanted to get back up to mom’s room, and it was lonely to eat by yourself anyway, so I just grabbed a banana and a granola bar. They had a pan of golden pancakes, tempting me with their scent, but I didn’t want to mess with syrup. I wasn’t sure how pancakes became a breakfast food, because by the time you poured syrup over them, they might as well be a dessert. But they were delicious!

I got back up to the ICU doors and hesitated, looking for the phone to call in. I didn't see one there, so I just tried pushing on the door and it opened. I stepped through gingerly, hoping it was okay to just walk in. I was used to the ICU being locked and having to call in for permission to enter. Maybe they hadn't bothered with that here, since they didn't use the unit that often.

Gina and another lady were standing in mom's room, next to her bed. The other lady had fine, dark brown hair that was held off her face by a pink cloth headband. She had reading glasses on a chain around her neck and she was listening intently to what Gina was telling her. Mom was awake and listening also, so I figured it was okay if I went in the room. Sometimes, nurses need to tell stuff to other staff that we don't really want the family to hear. Usually it's stuff about the family that's not so flattering. I hoped that wasn't the case today!

I walked in and stood off to the side, as Gina finished telling the day nurse about mom's night. Mom looked over at me and smiled, which made the nurses turn around.

"This is Rhonda, the day nurse," Gina said. She looked really tired now, and I'm sure she was glad to be done with this impromptu night shift.

"I'm Allie, her daughter," I introduced myself to Rhonda. "I hope it's okay that I just came back in. There wasn't a phone to call."

Rhonda smiled at that. "It's fine," she said. "We've never had a secured door, mostly because we rarely use this unit."

I set my coffee and breakfast on the side counter as Rhonda completed her assessment. Mom's vital signs still looked good, and she seemed fairly comfortable when she was just resting in the bed. I settled into the recliner and peeled my banana. I couldn't think of anything else to do, so eating seemed to be the best use of my time.

Rhonda finished asking mom about pain and how she was breathing, and then told her that a breakfast tray would come shortly and she could eat breakfast. Mom nodded and Rhonda made sure the bedside table was next to the bed and within arms' reach. Then she walked back out to the desk and started charting. I wondered if this was all the day would entail. That was fine with me, but it would be a long, boring 12-hour shift if you only had one patient and they didn't need much.

I finished my banana and granola bar and was most of the way through my coffee when my phone buzzed in my pocket.

'*How is everything this morning?*' Jake wanted to know. It was almost 8, so he was just getting off shift.

'*She threw a PE last night. In the ICU. Can't transfer out b/c of the weather,*' I replied. After I hit 'send' I realized that sounded a bit dramatic, so I hastily sent another message. '*Doing ok, on O2 mask, but awake.*'

A few seconds later, my phone rang, and I didn't have to look at the screen to see who it was. I tried to answer as nonchalantly as possible.

"What happened?" Jake asked.

"She was getting up to the bathroom a little before 3 in the morning, and she suddenly started having trouble breathing," I said. "They put her on O2 by mask, and transferred her to the ICU."

"Madison has an ICU?" Jake said, skeptically.

"Yes, a small one," I replied. I didn't want to say anything derogatory about the unit because it was doing the job we needed, and besides, it was all we had.

"Normally, they would transfer her out, but we're snowed in," I continued. "So we're going to hang out and hope for the best. She's okay when she's resting, but any kind of activity really makes her breathe hard."

"Wow, that's kinda scary," Jake said. "How are you holding up?"

I chuckled softly, and said, "Honestly, better than I would've thought."

"That's good," Jake replied. "Found some new secret meditation technique?"

I could hear the mirth in his voice. I was not known for staying calm and unworried, especially in situations like this.

"Actually, I found a Bible and it had a bookmark on the exact page that I needed," I confessed. "I was a lot more peaceful after I read that."

"Well, good," Jake said. "God's watching out for you."

I knew God was always watching out for me, but sometimes I needed little reminders of it. So first God had to take care of me, and then He had to keep reminding me that He was taking care of me. I kept Him busy, I guess.

"So, what's the plan now?" Jake asked.

"She's on the injections for the blood clot," I replied. "We're just going to stay here and keep her oxygen level up while her body breaks down the clot. No one really knows how long that will take."

"I guess you can't drive home anyway, huh?" he said.

"Nope," I laughed. "The road is closed and I'm stuck here for awhile."

"What are you going to do to keep from going crazy?" Jake wanted to know. I wasn't really the kind of person to sit around, and there wasn't much for entertainment here.

"Not sure," I sighed. "I'm going to look for a book to read. Maybe I should go see if I can help out in their ER," I joked.

"Well, they would probably love to have you," he agreed, "but then they would want you to stay there, and I don't want you to stay in Madison. I want you to come back to Brighton."

"Why is that?" I asked, thinking something must be up at work.

"Because I miss you," Jake said, earnestly. My heart skipped a beat and I had no idea how to reply to that. I usually dismissed these comments as Jake just joking around, but he didn't sound like he was joking.

"I promise I won't get a job in Madison," I told him. "I'll be back as soon as mom gets out of ICU and the road opens."

"Good," he replied. "Call me later when you're going bonkers and I'll distract you for awhile."

I promised I would call him later and disconnected. Of course, I didn't need to be on the phone with Jake for him to distract me. My mind kept wandering back over the conversation and replaying the part where Jake said he missed me.

Mom's breakfast tray had arrived and she was sitting up in the bed, eating. They had taken off her oxygen mask so she could eat, and had put the cannula on her nose instead. Even the effort of eating was making her breathe harder. I could tell she was hungry, but I didn't know how much she would get eaten before she was too worn out to finish.

Dad had finally woke up and wandered back in to the ICU. He snagged a piece of toast off mom's tray and munched on it. I didn't protest, because mom wasn't going to finish the meal anyway, no point in the food going to waste.

I sent a quick text to the other kids telling them nothing had changed. We hadn't seen Dr. Lytle yet, but he was up pretty late last night. Or early this morning, however you wanted to look at it. I was confident that Rhonda would call him if anything was out of the ordinary, and right now, nothing was.

I walked out to the desk to ask about finding a book. I knew there was a stash of reading material somewhere, every hospital had one. It got used mostly by night shift workers, but occasionally a bored patient or family member used it as well.

Rhonda was on the phone when I walked up to the desk, so I turned around to walk back into mom's room. Standing at the desk, listening in on the conversation was rude, and I always hated it when visitors did that to me. Especially if I was trying to talk to someone about a patient or some other private matter.

"Ok, Dr. Lytle, we'll see you later," I heard Rhonda say and hang up the phone. I turned back around toward the desk.

"Dr. Lytle was just checking in on Betty," Rhonda explained. "He'll be in later for rounds."

"Ok," I replied. "I'm looking for a book to read. Do you have anything around here?"

"Oh, honey, we have lots of entertainment around here," Rhonda laughed. She motioned me to come with her around the back of the desk and into their small break room area. There was a full size book case in there that had books, crossword puzzles, Sudoku, card games and puzzles stacked on it.

"ICU is a little boring here," she said. "We usually only have one patient, so we have to entertain ourselves."

"How did you end up working in the ICU here?" I asked her.

"I worked a cardiac unit years ago, when we lived in Texas," she explained. "We moved here when my husband's father died and he inherited the family business. There wasn't anything close to a cardiac unit here, but I had ICU experience, so they asked me to be part of the pool. There's about four of us that all have ICU in our background somewhere. We take turns covering call, and about eighty percent of the time, we never get called."

I was impressed that this small town hospital had such a good supply of critical care nurses. Even though the patients here weren't that critical, I had noticed that both of the nurses so far were very particular about my mom's care. They paid attention to every detail and checked on her frequently. Some things were just ingrained in certain nurses, and they never left, no matter how long they had been out of the game.

"Help yourself to whatever you want," Rhonda gestured at the book case. I thanked her and turned to see what my options were. I didn't really like puzzles of any kind, I got too frustrated with them. I did love to read though, so I started browsing the dozens of books on the shelf.

I skipped past some gory murder mystery books, as well as a few psychological thrillers. I was looking for something to relax me, not make me jumpier. One cover caught my eye with the title *Someone to Bring Her Flowers*, and I chuckled as I remembered Emmilynn's admonition that a man who brings flowers is a keeper. This book was a romance, though, and a pretty cheesy-looking one at that. I kept browsing for something a little more entertaining and finally settled on a Nicholas Sparks novel.

I walked back to mom's room and settled into the chair, since dad was kicked back in the recliner. It was like we had this fun little game of musical chairs going on, whenever someone got up, the other one took the recliner.

Fifteen minutes later my butt was already numb. This chair was not the least bit comfortable, and the book was good, but not good enough to distract me from how uncomfortable I was. I decided I would go check out the couch in the waiting room. Mom was dozing in the bed and nothing was going on. I told dad where I was going and headed down the hall to the little waiting room. It was empty, as I had expected, since we were the only people in the ICU.

The couch was surprisingly comfortable, and I didn't have to share the room with anyone, so I kicked my feet up and stretched out the length of the couch. I opened the book and got lost in the story.

Someone walking by the door of the waiting room caught my eye, and I looked up to see Dr. Lytle headed down the hall to the ICU. I was surprised to see that an hour had gone past already. What a difference a not-numb butt made.

I jumped up and followed Dr. Lytle into the unit. He went to the desk first to talk to Rhonda so I went in to mom's room to wait for him to come in. Mom was still dozing and dad was watching a hunting show on TV. Everything looked pretty status quo and I felt confident we just had to ride this out and mom would be fine.

Dr. Lytle came in to see mom after a few minutes, and he seemed to feel the same. Nothing was too far out of whack, and mom looked good.

"Betty, I wish this hadn't happened, but it looks like it will all work out," he said, smiling. "You sure gave me a run for my money, though!"

"I didn't mean to cause you any trouble," mom started to apologize, but Dr. Lytle waved her off.

"No, no, it wasn't anything you could control," he assured her. "And it's good for someone to keep me on my toes.

"Although," he continued, "consider your work done." He scowled at mom seriously for a moment before breaking into a grin. Mom smiled back at him and dad and I chuckled. It was good to relax and laugh, it made it feel like everything was normal again.

Dr. Lytle told mom he would check back on her later, after he rounded on the rest of his patients in the hospital. He walked out to the desk and sat down to write in her chart.

"I need to use the bathroom again," mom told me. I wasn't completely sure how to finagle her monitor wires, so I pressed the call light for Rhonda. I had been happy to help my mom when she was in the regular hospital room, but she had a lot more stuff stuck to her now.

Rhonda came right in, probably thankful to have something to do for a few minutes. She still wanted mom to use the bedside commode instead of walking to the bathroom, so dad and I stepped out. Rhonda told us we could just wait in the hallway until mom was done.

We walked out and stood in the hall, looking around the small unit. There were three patient rooms, but one looked like it was being used for storage. It had a random assortment of wheelchairs, small tables, boxes and a jumble of plastic tubes. I saw a ventilator tucked in one corner, and it looked like it was about 30 years old. I imagine they didn't see any need to buy a new one, since they didn't keep people here that needed to be on a ventilator.

I was standing there, lost in thought, when the monitor suddenly started alarming loudly. I jumped a little, but I knew the monitors frequently alarm when the patient is moving. I didn't panic, at least not at first. Then I heard Rhonda call out,

"Dr. Lytle!" with a touch of panic in her voice. And then I started to panic. Dr. Lytle had looked over at the monitor screen sitting on the nurses' desk when the alarm first rang and he was already up and running into the room.

Somewhere in my brain, my logical ER nurse side said ‘don’t go in the room, you’ll just be in the way,’ but it got drowned out by the daughter side that said ‘that’s my mom in there!’

I walked just to the door and looked in past the curtain that Rhonda had drawn across the door. Mom was sitting on the commode still, looking very pale, and the cardiac monitor showed her heart rate was 146. I could see from the door that the pattern was irregular now and the monitor was still dinging loudly.

“Betty, are you ok?” he asked mom, who was staring straight ahead and swaying slightly. Rhonda pressed the button to measure a blood pressure reading, and then realized she had disconnected the cuff when mom transferred to the commode. She was standing next to mom, holding on to her so she didn’t fall over, and she didn’t want to step away. My nurse mode kicked back in and I walked quickly to the bedside.

“Here, I’ll get the cuff,” I said, grabbing the cable and reaching over the bed to connect it to the cuff still on mom’s arm. I got it connected and Rhonda pressed the button again.

“Thank you!” Rhonda said to me, looking extremely grateful. It suddenly struck me how isolated we were in this tiny little unit so far away from the rest of the hospital. She didn’t really have a way to call out for help.

“Her O2 sat,” Rhonda said, gesturing at the other cable laying on the bed. She had taken the little clip off mom’s finger so she could move easier, but now we needed it back on so we could monitor mom’s condition. I grabbed the clip and slipped it on to my mom’s finger, noting how cool her skin felt. I focused hard on the task, to keep from getting too emotional. I needed to keep it together, my mom needed me and I didn't do her any good if I was a blubbering mess.

The monitor beeped once that the blood pressure had registered and the number flashing on the screen was '89/49'. My heart plummeted. Her heart rate was still fluctuating from 140 to 150, and her oxygen level was only 90%. Her face was still pale and she just generally did not look very good.

"We need to get her back on the bed," Dr. Lytle said. If she was laying down, her blood pressure would improve, since her heart wouldn't have to pump against gravity. Unfortunately, mom didn't look like she was going to be able to stand and transfer back to the bed. Luckily, I had a lot of experience with helping someone who could barely stand get from one place to the other, and I think Rhonda did too. We quickly moved into position on either side of mom and reached to hold her under each arm.

"On three," Rhonda said, and then counted 'one, two, three' and we smoothly pulled mom up to a standing position and then pivoted her and set her back down on the edge of the bed. Rhonda pulled the commode out of the way and reached down for mom's legs, swinging them up onto the bed as I guided her shoulders into the center of the bed. In five quick seconds, mom was now laying down in the bed, still looking pale but now we didn't have to worry about her falling over.

I stepped back out of the way and stood by dad, who was watching the whole scene nervously. I wanted to reassure him, but I didn't really have anything to say.

“Miles from home and you still get put to work, huh?” dad joked weakly. I had joked to Jake that I was going to work here to keep myself entertained.

But I didn’t mean it!

Chapter Fourteen

"We need a 12-lead," Dr. Lytle said to Rhonda. "It looks like a-fib with RVR."

Rhonda nodded and walked quickly out to the desk, where she retrieved the ECG machine and wheeled it back into the room. This was something I was familiar with, we did them in the ER all the time. It took three times as long to set up the machine and connect the wires as it did to take the actual reading, so we always did it as a team. Instinct kicked in and I stepped back up to the bed.

"I can do the wires for you," I said to Rhonda, who looked relieved at the offer.

"Thanks," she said, handing me the sheet of stickers and the box with all the wires connected to it. This required me to get a little up close and personal with my mom, but I knew we needed this done as quickly as possible. I placed all the stickers and connected the wires, just as Rhonda finished putting in the information for the machine to take the reading. We stood back for the required ten seconds while the ECG read her heart rhythm, and then stared expectantly at the paper as it printed out. The monitor agreed with Dr. Lytle's diagnosis, and the top line read "Atrial Fibrillation, Rapid Ventricular Response". Rhonda tore it off and handed it to Dr. Lytle, who glanced at it and nodded.

Rhonda pressed the button to check another blood pressure reading. Her heart rate was still over 140, and when the monitor beeped with the blood pressure, it was flashing 93/53. Not much improvement from when she was sitting up.

To say that Dr. Lytle looked concerned would be an understatement. His face was a mixture of worry, indecision, and fear. I knew he was a good surgeon and I trusted him, but I had a feeling we had wandered out of his area of expertise. He appeared to be racking his brain for what he was supposed to do next.

"Rhonda, let's draw some blood and check cardiac enzymes," he said, sounding relieved that he had remembered something. "We'll repeat the d-dimer and a chest x-ray as well."

Rhonda nodded and walked out to a cupboard in the hallway that contained medical supplies. She returned with the necessary supplies and put the tourniquet on mom's arm. About then, the desk phone started ringing. Rhonda looked up briefly, but it was obvious she intended to keep on with patient care instead of letting the phone interrupt. I didn't think it was possible to like Rhonda even more, but right then, she was my favorite person in the whole world. A nurse who thought my mom was more important than a phone was a rare gift.

"I can answer that," I offered, partly to be nice, and partly because it was annoying me.

"Sure," Rhonda said, focused on the needle she was about to stick into my mom's vein. Dad had already slid back out into the hallway as soon as he had realized they were going to be poking my mom.

I walked out to the desk, picked up the phone, and said politely, “ICU, how can I help you?”

“This is Karen,” said a voice I recognized as the house supervisor I had met on Monday. She had a touch of a question in her tone, probably because she didn’t recognize the voice answering.

“Hi Karen, it’s Allie, Betty Sanford’s daughter,” I hastily explained. “Rhonda is busy in with mom so I said I would answer the phone.”

“Oh, ok,” she said. “How is Betty doing?”

“She went in to a-fib, and her pressure dropped,” I said, calmly. I kept pretending to myself that this wasn’t my mom, but just some random patient we were talking about. That made it easier to stay emotionally detached.

“Oh no!” Karen cried. “I’ll be right there.”

I heard the phone clatter down so I knew she had hung up, and I imagined she was quickly striding toward the ICU right now. I set the phone back in the cradle and went into the room to tell Rhonda that Karen was on her way.

Rhonda looked relieved that she was going to have another nurse on hand to help out. I had been in her shoes before, trying to manage everything alone, and it was frustrating. There are so many things that have to be done in such a short period of time.

Rhonda finished drawing the blood and wrapped the bandage around mom's arm. Dr. Lytle had been listening to mom's heart and lungs with his stethoscope, and he still looked fairly unsure of himself.

Karen came walking quickly into the unit and immediately asked Rhonda what she needed. Rhonda handed her the tubes of blood and said they needed taken to lab. Karen nodded and walked off again. Rhonda went out to the desk to call x-ray and have them come take the chest x-ray.

Dr. Lytle walked over where I was standing, near the door. Dad was still out in the hallway, but the unit was so small, he was only about eight feet away.

"Allie, Bob, I have to be honest with you," he said apologetically, "I'm in a little over my head now. This isn't something I've ever had to deal with before."

He looked at me, almost pleadingly. "I know I should know what to do, I'm sure I learned it somewhere in residency. But I can't remember and I don't want to guess."

I admired his honesty with me and I fervently agreed that he shouldn't be guessing at what to do. An important lesson I had to learn in nursing school was to admit when you don't know something. Don't try to wing it- people end up dead that way.

Suddenly, a thought popped in my head, so abruptly I swear I actually heard a popping noise.

"Wait, there's this one thing that Dr. Raymond is always talking about," I burst out, my words tumbling over each other. "There's a university and their medical department does a remote consult, and they can look at everything over a video stream! They tell you what you should do. He told us about it in Brighton. He wants us to use it but he can't convince any of the doctors to try it."

Dr. Lytle looked at me, startled. "I remember hearing about that at a conference last year," he said. "I've never seen anyone use it. How would it work from here?"

"Well, I'll need to look it up for sure," I said, "and we need a way to video call them." I deflated slightly as I realized that Madison Hospital probably wouldn't have the technology we needed.

"I can do that," Dr. Lytle said, and gestured for me to follow him to the desk. He pulled a tablet computer out of his bag and touched the screen to light it up. "I use this for video calls all the time. Mostly with my mom," he added, sheepishly. "What's the name of the university?"

I told him the information that I knew, thankful that I had listened to Dr. Raymond at least one of the times he was talking about this. At the time, I was probably just being polite, because he talked about it a lot. He was adamant that this was the future of rural medicine, and right now, I could see his point.

Dr. Lytle got to the webpage, and there was a link right there that said “Call now”. He clicked on it, and symbol of a ringing phone started dancing on the screen.

The dancing phone was suddenly replaced by the face of a young Asian man. He was wearing wire rim glass and a white lab coat, and he looked like he was about twenty years old. He was obviously older than that if he was working in a medical department, but he still looked young. I couldn’t imagine he was the guy who was going to be our professional consult.

“University Telemedicine,” he said politely, with a trace of an accent. “Are you in need of a medical consult?”

“Yes, I am,” Dr. Lytle said fervently, as if he needed to convince the young man to help him.

“What specialty?” the young man asked, politely. I breathed a sigh of relief when I realized he was just the guy who answers the phone. That made sense, cardiologists don’t want to sit around and answer random phone calls. I was just jittery and jumping to conclusions.

“Cardiology or pulmonology,” Dr. Lytle said. “I have a patient with a PE who went into a-fib.”

“Ok, one moment, please,” the young man said, nodding as he talked. The screen flashed, went blank for a moment, and then flashed again. We were now looking at a man in his sixties, with thick bushy eyebrows and graying hair.

"Dr. Boding, Cardiology," he said in a deep authoritative voice. "What's the situation?"

Dr. Lytle filled him in on mom's condition and our rural location and weather status, adding that he really was out of his league trying to handle this problem.

"Fantastic!" Dr. Boding replied, enthusiastically. I was a bit surprised by that, because nothing about this situation seemed fantastic to me.

"This is precisely why we designed this program," he continued. "It's great to see it working!"

While I was glad he was excited to see it working, I wanted it to work a little quicker. Which was irrational on my part, we had a cardiologist on the case in under a minute. If we had had to call in a cardiologist, we would still be waiting for him to get there. Patience wasn't my strong suit.

"Ok, let's start at the top," he said, briskly. "Show me the ECG."

Dr. Lytle held up the red and white piece of paper so the camera was pointing at it. Dr. Boding looked at it for a long minute, making 'mm-hmm' noises to himself. Then he asked for her most current lab results and vital signs. He pondered those for a moment, making some notes on a paper, and then asked to see the original chest x-ray.

" It's in our digital imaging system," Dr. Lytle explained. Dr. Boding nodded, understandingly.

“If you pull up the image on your computer screen, then turn the camera toward it, I can usually see it pretty well,” he instructed.

Dr. Lytle did as he asked, and Dr. Boding looked at it carefully.

“We’re getting a repeat chest x-ray right now,” Dr. Lytle informed him.

“Good, good, that’s the best thing to do,” Dr. Boding said, and Dr. Lytle looked relieved and a little proud that he had remembered one of the things correctly.

“Ok, now let me see the patient,” Dr. Boding said. Dr. Lytle picked up his tablet and walked into mom’s room.

“Betty, this is Dr. Boding, a cardiologist at the university,” Dr. Lytle explained, pointing to the screen. Mom looked at his image inquisitively, as if she wasn’t sure why it was being shown to her.

“Betty, nice to meet you,” Dr. Boding spoke and mom visibly jumped. Apparently, she didn’t realize it was a live video stream. She looked a little frightened and unsure, so I hastened to reassure her.

“Mom, it’s a video feed of a cardiologist who can look over your case and help us decide how to treat you,” I explained to her. She looked at me cautiously, and then back to the video screen.

“Um, hello,” she said, tentatively.

Dr. Boding explained each step to Dr. Lytle, who first moved the tablet so the camera could look at mom's breathing pattern, then at her hands and feet, especially that left leg, then up to the monitor where her heart rhythm was being traced. He asked Dr. Lytle several questions about her lung sounds, and the quality of her pulses. Then he asked to talk to mom again, so Dr. Lytle placed the tablet in front of her.

"Betty, in general, how do you feel?" Dr. Boding asked.

"Fine, I guess," mom answered, seeming uncomfortable with talking to a computer screen. They had never done any kind of video calling, so this was foreign to her.

"Take a deep breath for me," Dr. Boding said, and mom complied, wincing slightly.

"Does it hurt to do that?" he asked.

"No, not really," mom answered, always the one to downplay her symptoms.

"Well, then why did you grimace?" Dr. Boding asked bluntly. Mom just shrugged, not sure how to reply.

"Betty, I'm sure this is weird," he said, softening. "Most people in a small town are used to being seen by a doctor that's known them forever and they feel comfortable with him. Nobody wants to be seen by a guy they don't know, who isn't even in the room. It feels weird to talk to a computer screen with some guys head on it, I know. But since I can't be there, I need you to help me know what you're going through. So you need to tell me everything, and I mean everything, that you feel. Ok?"

Mom nodded, glancing at me, nervously.

"It's okay, mom, you'll do fine," I patted her hand as I reassured her.

"And who is this lovely young lady?" Dr. Boding asked, jovially.

"This is my daughter, Allison," mom said proudly. "She's an ER nurse."

I smiled and waved a couple fingers at the video camera.

"Well, she obviously gets her looks from you," Dr. Boding said. "Who does she get her brains from?" he asked, jokingly.

"That's a mix of her dad and me," mom answered. "She gets her practical side from her dad, that's for sure. I could never do what she does!"

"It's always nice to have a nurse around, isn't it?" Dr. Boding said.

"Oh, she's been just wonderful," mom gushed. "She came over here the night before surgery and she took the entire week off work to stay with me. She's a wonderful daughter, I don't know what we would do without her."

While I certainly didn't mind hearing my mom say how wonderful I was, I thought this conversation had gotten a bit off track. Just about then, Dr. Boding turned his questions back to my mom's medical condition.

As he asked her more questions about the pain, and where and when she felt it, asking her to describe it in detail, I noticed she was much more relaxed and answered his questions thoroughly. Ahh, well played, Dr. Boding. Getting mom to talk about her daughter made her relax enough to be willing to talk about her symptoms. Perhaps our cardiologist had minored in psychology. If you want a mom to talk, just ask her about her kids.

As Dr. Boding was finishing up his questions with my mom, Rhonda stuck her head in the door to tell Dr. Lytle that the lab results and x-ray were back. He took his tablet with Dr. Boding's head on it out to the desk with him, telling us he would be back shortly.

"That was odd," mom said to me. "Had you ever seen that before?"

"Actually, it was my idea," I told her. "We have a doctor at work who is always talking about telemedicine. He says it's the future of rural medicine and that we don't have to always send our patients out, we can treat them in our hometown, and just get expert consultation over the internet. I usually didn't pay much attention to him, but something must have stuck in my brain, because when Dr. Lytle told me he didn't know what to do for you, I suddenly remembered this website."

“Do you know this doctor we just talked to?” mom asked me. I shook my head.

“They have specialists at the medical university that are available for whatever specialty you need,” I explained. “Honestly, I don’t know everything about it, so maybe I’ll have to listen a little closer next time Dr. Raymond is talking about it.”

Dr. Raymond would probably be even more ecstatic than Dr. Boding had been when he found out that we had used his precious telemedicine to help my mom. And I had to agree, she made a pretty good case for using it.

Dr. Lytle came back in, without his tablet, but holding a slip of paper he had written some orders on.

“We discussed the options for trying to get your heart back in a normal rhythm,” he said. “Cardioversion isn’t an option without more cardiac support than what we can provide here. Medication is the next choice, and given your pulmonary status, we will err on the side of caution and use a diltiazem drip.”

He looked at me more than once as he explained that, and I knew most of those details were for my benefit. My parents didn’t really know what all those things were, but I was glad he broke down the decision process. Obviously, Dr. Boding had been very thorough in considering all the aspects of my mom’s condition.

Rhonda was walking in with a small plastic bag of clear IV fluid and some IV tubing, which I assumed was the diltiazem. She set up the pump as Dr. Lytle finished talking.

“We will watch your heart rate, and your blood pressure, to see how this is working, and re-evaluate in two hours. I’ll call Dr. Boding back sooner if something happens.”

Rhonda connected the IV and started the pump. She messed with the cardiac monitor for a moment, and then turned and said, “That blood pressure cuff will go off every fifteen minutes now. Tell me right away if anything feels out of the ordinary.”

Mom said she would, and Rhonda went back out to the desk.

“Does anyone have any questions?” Dr. Lytle wanted to know. All three of us shook our heads. “Allie, you really came to the rescue today,” he said, earnestly. “I don’t know what I would have done without you.”

“God always puts her right where she needs to be, I’ve noticed,” my dad commented. Dr. Lytle laughed and agreed with him. He promised us he would be back in thirty minutes to check on mom, and headed out the door.

I just sat there, staring at mom for a long moment. She looked pale and completely exhausted. I had seen a hundred other patients looking like this, but seeing it on my own mom was totally different. A pain stabbed through my heart and I wished, once again, that I could just take this away from her.

I glanced over at my dad, and he was watching me, searching my face for signs of worry. I guess I was his barometer for deciding how bad off mom was. Truthfully, it wasn't as bad as it could have been. We had gotten the help we needed, and the really scary part was over. But I had grown wary of deciding we were in the clear now, because I had decided that twice in the last two days, and I was wrong both times.

What if something worse happened? What if we needed a piece of equipment that they didn't have here? They had a 30-year-old ventilator, which wasn't that reassuring. My worrywart side was starting to get really revved up as my mind started spinning through all the possible things that could go wrong.

Mom coughed and readjusted herself in the bed, and that minor distraction derailed my worry train, at least for now. I realized I hadn't called Shelby or Andrew with the latest development, so I reached for my phone with a sigh. I decided I would go out to the waiting room to make the calls, since mom looked like she was resting.

I dialed Shelby as I walked down the hall. She was probably at work now, and I wasn't sure how much information to leave on her voicemail. Some things just needed to be said in person and not heard in a message.

Sure enough, I got voice mail. I left a generic message saying I needed to update her on mom and she should call me as soon as possible. I tried to sound calm, so she wouldn't get too worried. I called Andrew next, who answered on the first ring. Did he just keep his phone in his hand? Most of the time, by the time I realized my phone was ringing and then located it, the person had already hung up.

"How's she doing, sis?" he asked, skipping past the polite conversation.

"She had another setback," I started out. "Her heart went into a really fast, irregular rate, and they started her on an IV medication to try to get it back to normal. We're going to wait two hours and see how she does."

That seemed like a very brief synopsis of everything that had happened in the last hour, but most of the details didn't really matter, at least for Andrew.

"What now?" he wanted to know. Ah, there was that question again. I was asking it myself, and I sure didn't have an answer for everyone else. Luckily, being a nurse trains you for this. Patients and families are constantly asking questions you didn't have the answer to. You learned how to give an answer that didn't really say anything.

"A cardiologist is consulting over a video stream, and we will check back with him after two hours," I replied. "Then he'll decide what course of action to take."

Didn't that sound good? We still didn't have an answer, other than *wait and see.* Which was one of my least favorite answers, but it was the only one we had.

"Can I talk to her?" Andrew asked. Apparently, hearing her voice helped assure him she was ok. I could understand that.

"She's really wiped out and she's resting right now," I said, apologetically. "How about if we call you in about an hour, after she gets a nap?"

He agreed to that and said he would keep the phone close by. I decided to send an update text to Lacey and Jake, since they had both been concerned about mom. I didn't want to make people worry, but they would both understand what was going on.

I noticed my book still laying on the side table, where I had set it down when I got up to follow Dr. Lytle into the ICU. That felt like it had been days ago, even though it had been less than two hours. I had to stop and think for a minute what the book was even about, and then I decided I might as well sit and read for a bit, since mom was sleeping.

I had only read a few pages, when my phone buzzed with a text message. I looked at the screen and fought a smile when I saw it was from Jake.

'That's not great news. Has the weather let up?' he asked.

I hadn't even looked out a window yet today, so I honestly didn't know what the weather looked like. Even if it had stopped snowing, it would take a while before the town got shoveled out from under all that snow.

'Haven't looked recently. I hope she turns around after this,' I replied.

'It quit snowing here this morning,' his next message read.

'And I've been shoveling snow for 4 hrs!' was the message that followed. I laughed at that, because I had done my share of snow shoveling as well. Someday I was going to move south where it never snowed and I never had to bundle up before the sun came up and go clear off my sidewalk. This blizzard was one of those snowstorms where you shoveled every few hours, even though it was still snowing, or else there was more snow than you could move with a shovel. My little house was going to be buried.

'It's good cardio. Builds upper body strength,' I texted back, adding a smiley face. Jake liked to work out a lot, but I think he preferred a gym. Honestly, I didn't know anyone who liked to shovel snow.

'Yeah, good thing I'm so strong,' he replied.

'See, those muscles are good for more than just looks!' I texted. After I hit send, I realized that sounded a little, well, gushing bunker bunny. I mean, Jake looked good and everyone knew it. I just didn't mean to come across like that.

'Miss Allie, you make me blush! I didn't know you even noticed my muscles,' his message said. Right. I would have to be dead not to notice his muscles. Even if I was blind, I could still feel them when he put his arm around my shoulders.

The guys at the fire department like to make jokes about 'Body by Jake', but Jake didn't look like the overgrown, no-neck, bodybuilder type. He wasn't much bigger than other guys his height, but he was fitter than most of them. The dark blue t-shirts they wore as their uniform hugged tightly to his shoulders and showed off the curve of his bicep. I didn't like to think I was shallow when it came to what I found attractive in a man, but Jake's physique was definitely one of his assets.

He was more than just a pretty face, though. Jake was one of the nicest people I knew, and I wasn't the only one who thought so. Everybody liked Jake. He brought a positive energy into the room with his easygoing demeanor and infectious smile. He truly cared about people and was always willing to help someone out. Working as paramedic really let him shine as caregiver and provider.

But Jake and I were just friends. I mean, I had certainly wondered what it would feel like to be wrapped in his strong arms, but I always reminded myself that there were about a hundred women who would love to be in Jake's arms. We were good friends, and I didn't want it to get all weird and awkward if I developed a crush on him. While all the teasing and flirting was fun, I never took it too seriously. I didn't even know if Jake had ever thought of me as more than just a friend.

My phone rang, startling me out of my thoughts. It was Shelby, calling me back, which snapped me back to reality.

"Hey," I answered.

"What happened?" Shelby asked, which was becoming her normal way of answering the phone.

I filled her in on mom's heart rhythm problems and the new IV medication. Shelby giggled a little at hearing how mom reacted to talking to a computer screen.

"I'm surprised they don't do video calling with Andrew's girls," she commented.

"Their computer doesn't have a camera," I reminded her. "Maybe we should get them one for Christmas. Then they could see the girls more."

"Good idea, 'Lis," Shelby said, enthusiastically. "You pick it out and tell me how much I owe."

I had been down this road before. I bought the present, wrapped it, picked out the card and then Shelby conveniently forgot to ever pay me for her half. I was used to it by now. Looks like I was buying my parents a camera for their computer. At least I had one gift checked off my shopping list.

"I heard it quit snowing there," I changed the subject, to avoid the argument.

"Yep. The streets are mostly plowed by now, but the sidewalks are still pretty buried, so getting around is a little tricky."

I was imagining my little house buried in snow and dreading the snow removal task I had waiting for me when

I got back, when Shelby asked, "Who did you hire to do your walks?"

"What do you mean?" I asked.

"Who shovels your sidewalks?" she asked, again.

"I do!" I replied, laughing.

"Well, you didn't do them today, and they're all cleared off," she informed me, tartly.

"They are?" I asked, incredulously.

"Yeah, I drove by on my way to work, just to check on your house, and you have the cleanest sidewalk on the street," she replied.

"Well, maybe the neighbor did it," I guessed. "Jim and Cathy know I'm out of town."

"Except their walk is still buried," Shelby added. "I thought you had hired a snow removal service."

"Nope," I replied, still perplexed at who would have shoveled off my walk for me. Especially if it wasn't Jim.

I remembered Jake saying he had been shoveling snow for hours. That obviously involved more snow than just his own sidewalk, but I hadn't really thought about where he was shoveling. Had he really driven all the way to my house to shovel my sidewalks while I was out of town?

That would be a good friend, indeed.

Chapter Fifteen

I hung up with Shelby, still wondering about Jake and my sidewalk. I couldn't get focused on the book again, so I went back into the ICU to check on mom.

She was sitting up in the bed and looked a little more alert. She smiled at me when I walked in, which was reassuring to see. She had looked pretty rough earlier. I sneaked a glance at the cardiac monitor and saw that her heart rate was still irregular, but was now only 100 and her blood pressure was 105/65. That was better.

"How are you feeling, mom?" I said.

"Better," she replied. "I had a nice nap."

"Do you feel up to talking on the phone?" I asked her.

"Oh, sure!" she said, cheerfully. She must have guessed she was going to talk to Andrew, which meant she got to talk to Cassie and Sammie too. Her phone was in the drawer still but I didn't know how much battery was left, so I just pulled mine out of my pocket, hit Andrew's name and handed her the phone.

"I told him everything that happened," I explained to her. "He just wanted to talk to you."

She nodded and a moment later, started talking to Andrew. I looked over at dad, who was watching something on a sports channel. My stomach growled, reminding me that breakfast was a long time ago.

"Dad, are you hungry?" I asked him.

"Yep," he replied. "I was just thinking about getting some lunch."

Since mom was busy on the phone, we just waved to her and headed for the cafeteria. Rhonda and Karen were sitting at the desk, chatting. I was grateful for Karen hanging around the ICU, just in case they needed her help. I was glad to jump in, but I wasn't an ICU nurse, and there was only so much I could do.

We walked in to the cafeteria and were met with the delicious aroma of Italian food. Lasagna was on the menu today, and I hoped it tasted as good as it smelled. Now that I smelled food, I was ravenous.

We got our plates and found a table to sit at. I dug into my food with gusto. The lasagna was good, but not as good as Tony's Italian food. Luckily, I wasn't a picky eater, at least not when I was this hungry. I finished my food in record time.

Dad was still eating, but he wasn't far behind me. He had only eaten a piece of toast off mom's breakfast tray, which made my granola bar and banana look like a full meal. After the adrenaline rush from all this morning's events, we both needed some fuel in the tank.

Dad finished up and we headed back to mom's room. There was this unspoken concern about being gone for too long, even though our presence there wasn't going to stop anything else from happening. We both just wanted to be close by.

Mom was off the phone but still had a smile lingering on her face, so she must have been talking to the twins. They always seemed to have that effect on her. It was nice to see her looking happy, it made her look better overall. Her heart rate was still hanging around 100 and the diltiazem wasn't working its magic so far- her heartbeat was still irregular.

"How was lunch?" she asked us.

"Good," dad replied. "Lasagna. Not as good as yours, though." Mom smiled sweetly at him when he said that.

"Have you talked to Shelby?" mom asked me. It was assumed that I was going to be the one updating the family. Dad didn't seem too keen to take on the role, and it did make more sense for me to do it, since I knew the most about what was going on.

"Yeah, I talked to her about an hour ago," I replied. "She's at work today. It quit snowing there this morning."

"It's clearing out here, too," dad remarked. I had noticed that the sun was shining now, but the outside world was still buried in a thick blanket of white. At least the plows and snow shovels could catch up now that it had stopped snowing.

We sat around making small talk for thirty minutes. The general atmosphere in the room was relaxed, now that the situation didn't look so serious. We had been on a roller coaster for the last two days, and I was starting to feel a little wrung out.

Dr. Lytle walked in to the room as we were chatting. "You look good, Betty," he told mom. He frowned slightly at the cardiac monitor and I knew he was thinking the same thing I had- the diltiazem wasn't working. Her heart rate was down but her rhythm wasn't back to normal. However, her oxygen level and blood pressure looked better.

"I'm going to call Dr. Boding back and check in," Dr. Lytle told us. The plan was to check back in after two hours, to update Dr. Boding and re-evaluate the plan. I had really hoped the update would be a little more positive. It seemed we were going to get more '*wait and see*'.

Dr. Lytle went out to the desk to get his tablet and make the call. I felt nervous, but I didn't know why, really. I scrolled through my phone to distract myself, even though I wasn't seeing a single thing on the screen.

Dr. Lytle came back in, carrying the tablet with Dr. Boding's head on it. This time around, mom chatted with him easily. She didn't have much to say, she felt about the same as before. She hadn't tried getting out of bed again, so she wasn't having much trouble breathing. I wasn't eager to see how the next bathroom break went.

After Dr. Boding had finished talking to mom, Dr. Lytle went back out to the desk to finish the phone call. I abandoned the phone and sat there, picking at my cuticles. It was something I did when I was bored or edgy. And right now, I wasn't bored. I could feel dad watching me, but I kept my head down, furiously digging at this one little piece of dead skin. I needed to focus my nervous energy on something, and this was the best thing I could find right now.

Dr. Lytle walked back in, rescuing my cuticles from getting picked completely off, and sat down on one of the empty chairs.

"Well, Betty, nothing has changed," he started out. "That wasn't what we were hoping for, though. The diltiazem doesn't seem to be working, and we don't want to leave you in this irregular rhythm, because there's risks associated with it."

Mom nodded slowly, looking at him intently. He rubbed the back of his neck and looked up at the monitor again, as if he were willing it to change to a normal heart rhythm.

"We're limited for what we can do here, as you know," he continued. "The road is still closed, but they're hoping to open it soon. If you can get to Springfield, they have a lot more options."

I had mixed emotions on that news. Mom was stable right now, and Springfield was 150 miles away, which was going to be a hassle for dad. But if she was in

Springfield, we wouldn't have to worry about not having the help we needed if something else went wrong.

Was something else going to go wrong? That was the question no one could answer. What if we went through all the trouble of an ambulance transfer and then her heart went back to normal and nothing else was needed? Two hours ago, I wouldn't have thought twice about it-transferring to Springfield would have been the obvious choice. But now we had managed to get through this far, and mom was stable, even if she wasn't completely better. The roads weren't open yet, and even after they were, they were still snow-packed and slippery. Was it worth the risk of getting in an accident?

"Obviously, we have to wait until the road is open," Dr. Lytle said, "but I wanted to start talking about what you want to do, so when the road is open, we've made a decision."

Mom nodded understandingly. She looked at dad and then at me and then back to Dr. Lytle.

"What do you recommend?" she asked him.

"From a medical standpoint, you should transfer," Dr. Lytle said. "But it is your choice, and sometimes there's more to consider than just the data in your hospital chart. You are still in a-fib, but you're stable. Springfield is a long way from home, and the transfer has some risk because of road conditions. I won't tell you that you have to transfer, I just want you to know the pros and cons of both choices."

"Ok," mom replied. "We'll talk it over and decide."

Dr. Lytle nodded and stood to leave. "If anything changes in your condition, I'll let you know if it changes my recommendation," he told mom, earnestly.

After he had left, dad moved up to sit by mom's bed. He reached out and took her hand and asked her, "What do you think, Betty?"

Mom sighed in response. "I don't know. It seems like we're doing fine here. I feel better now and they're doing a great job. Springfield is so far away," her voice trailed off in indecision. She looked over at me, the unspoken question in her eyes.

I didn't have an answer for her, though. I was as torn as she was, but I was expected to weigh in with my expert opinion. I knew my mom would probably do what I said she should, but I didn't want to talk my mom into something that was the wrong decision. I wasn't prepared to deal with that level of responsibility. Or guilt.

I liked decisions that are black and white. Or at least dark gray and light gray. I didn't have trouble doing the right thing, as long as I knew what the right thing was. This decision was a checkerboard, each answer could be really right or really wrong.

"I have no idea, mom," I confessed. "I really don't know which way to go."

They both looked a little surprised at that. I usually had a very strong opinion on what should be done, and I wasn't bashful about making that opinion known. It was unusual for me to be at a loss, at least when it came to medical things. But, no matter how many times I turned over the options in my mind, I couldn't come up with a clear answer.

It would be a little different if the weather was completely clear. I just kept remembering last winter, when the ambulance in Brighton ended up in the ditch on three different occasions. Mom was better off in the tiny, old ICU in Madison than she was in a snowdrift.

"Well, we don't have to decide right away," mom said. "The road isn't open yet, so we'll just wait for a little bit. There's no rush."

My mom was so calm and practical, sometimes. She seemed completely unfazed by all this. I wondered if she was stressing out on the inside, like I was. If so, she hid it a lot better than I did.

While I was mulling over the situation, mom announced she needed to use the commode again. I walked out to the desk, to let Rhonda know her help was needed.

"Oh boy," Rhonda said, when I told her. I knew what she meant. Getting up to the commode was what had started this whole thing in the first place. But we couldn't very well tell mom she wasn't allowed to go to the bathroom ever again.

Dad and I stood in the hallway, while Rhonda helped mom up. I slid over beside the nurses' station where I could see the monitor on the desk. I wanted to be able to see if Rhonda needed help, although I wasn't sure I could be the help she needed.

Mom's heart rate picked up as she was getting up, which was expected. The highest heart rate I saw was 128, which wasn't as high as it had been before, but still higher than it should be.

After a few minutes, Rhonda came out and told us we could go back in. Mom was resting back in bed, breathing a little bit harder than she had been before she got up, but not looking as wiped out as the last time.

That didn't really help the decision-making process any. We were still in this ambiguous state, where we couldn't quite decide how serious mom's condition was. I was getting frustrated, although I didn't have anyone to be upset with. That just made my frustration worse. I liked to have someone to get mad and yell at.

I realized I had to use the bathroom myself, so I went out into the hallway where the visitor bathrooms were located. The bathroom was as old as the ICU, complete with pink tile and a metal sink. It was frigid in there, apparently bathrooms didn't use to be heated. It took forever for the water to get warm too, and after sitting on cold porcelain, I really wanted to run my hands under some nice warm water.

As I walked back past the waiting room, I saw my book sitting on the table where I had left it earlier. I stopped and picked it up. I was sure I would be too distracted to read, but I didn't want to leave a mess.

Sometimes I was amazed at what people would leave in the waiting room when they left. Partially eaten food, wrappers, opened mail, even a dirty diaper. I guess they figured someone else should clean up after them.

Before I headed back in to mom's room, I pulled out my phone to check for messages. I had a text message from Lacey, sending mom get-well wishes. I scrolled through a couple other messages that weren't urgent and was about to put my phone away when it buzzed with another message.

'*I can't believe you haven't had to call me for a distraction yet,*' the message from Jake read. I decided that right then, Jake was just the distraction I needed, so I hit the little phone icon next to his name. I could feel myself getting wound up, and I needed to derail that worry train.

"Wow, it's like I think about you and you appear!" Jake joked when he answered the phone.

I laughed. "I forgot I had you available as a distraction until your text reminded me," I explained.

"And you're in need of a distraction?" Jake asked. "Or did you punch somebody and now you need bail money?"

"No, there's no one to punch," I told him. "Everything that's wrong is no one's fault, unless you blame Mother Nature." I filled him in on our current situation and wondering if we should transfer when we had the chance or wait and see how she did.

Jake had been in an ambulance when it hit black ice and went sliding into the ditch. He was in the back with the patient and he got knocked around a little, so he understood my concern about sending mom down that slippery road in an ambulance.

"That's a sticky spot to be in," he sympathized. "What does your mom think?"

"She sounded like she would rather stay here," I told him. "But I know she'll do whatever I tell her. She trusts me to do what's best for her. It's just that I don't *know* what's best for her, and I'm driving myself crazy, trying to figure it out."

"Crazy Allie. That has a nice ring to it," Jake teased me. I laughed, in spite of myself. Jake was always good at breaking the tension with a little humor.

"Just wait until I totally crack," I joked back. "I'll stop bathing and start wearing six sets of clothes at one time. Someday, you'll get a call to come extricate me from my house, that's filled with cats and chickens."

"Don't be ridiculous. That would never happen," Jake replied. "The cats would eat the chickens."

"True. Cats and ferrets then. Or maybe chickens and gerbils. And a hundred dead plants."

"At least six sets of clothes is better than naked," Jake replied. "Those are always awkward."

I knew he was speaking from experience, and I was glad that those ones were at least wrapped up in a blanket before I had to see them. The naked ones usually weren't sober or in their right mind, so they weren't too cooperative with the paramedics trying to help them.

"I promise not to swing at you," I told him. "Or try to bite you. No matter how crazy I get."

"Sounds good," he replied. "And I promise not to let the cops Tase you."

That was just an inside EMS joke, because the cops rarely Tased people, and certainly not for trying to bite the paramedics. But they all liked to joke about it, and that kept some people a little more cooperative.

I felt more relaxed after laughing and talking about something other than my mom. See? Jake was a great distraction. I was glad I had called him. I promised to keep him updated and hung up the phone.

I was sitting on the little couch and I just sat there for a minute, trying to process everything now that I wasn't so keyed up. I still couldn't reach a decision, so I sighed and stood up to go back in the ICU.

Nothing had changed in mom's room, and I was never so disappointed to see status quo. She wasn't worse, at least. I was trying to keep a positive outlook.

I let mom know that Lacey was wishing her a quick recovery. That made her smile, my parents loved Lacey.

Everybody loved Lacey, really. She was just too sweet and kind not to like.

I pulled mom's cell phone out and plugged it in. If she ended up going to Springfield, I wouldn't be with her while she transferred, and I wanted to make sure I had a way to stay in touch with her. The transfer actually brought a whole new batch of logistic problems. We had gone through this when my dad transferred from Madison to Springfield with his heart attack. Dad could ride in the ambulance with mom, but then they didn't have a car to get home. I could ride in the ambulance and dad could drive, but then how did I get back to my car? I had to work again on Monday, so I needed my car to get to Brighton.

I leaned my head back against the wall behind me and closed my eyes in frustration, feeling overwhelmed by it all. I stayed like that for a few minutes, hoping the whole situation might magically work itself out by the time I opened my eyes.

I sat back up after a few minutes, and a spasm shot through my neck from sitting with my head back like that. I remembered the guy in the waiting room who slept that way. I would have been paralyzed.

"I know you're over there, stewing," dad observed. "Come up with anything?"

"No," I said, forlornly. "No matter how I look at it, I still don't get an answer."

"Did you ask God about it?" dad asked me.

Oh, yeah. Ask God. Why didn't I ever remember that? I spent so much time and effort trying to figure things out by myself. And all I did was drive myself bonkers for no good reason. I was going to end up with an ulcer from all this worrying, but I always forgot I had the help I needed. I just had to ask.

Between the TV and the cardiac monitor, I felt too distracted to hear God. I told mom and dad I would be back, and walked back out to the waiting room. There, in the silence, I asked God to show me the right thing to do. I sat there quietly, waiting for the answer, but I didn't hear one. I racked my brain for some helpful verse that would guide me, but I couldn't think of one.

"Trust in the Lord with all your heart", but that didn't help. I was trying to trust in the Lord, but I didn't know which decision was the trusting one. I wished I had my parents' faith. They made it look so easy. They didn't doubt God or struggle with trying to fix things without His help.

Maybe that was the answer. Maybe I didn't need to be the expert opinion. If my parents could trust God, I should trust my parents. Instead of feeling the burden of making this decision for my mom, I should step back and let her make it for herself. I wasn't in charge of this situation, and I needed to stop acting like I was.

I felt a huge burden lift off my shoulders, and I knew I had heard God's answer. Trusting God meant trusting my mom. I breathed a sigh of relief and walked back into the ICU.

Dad was sitting by the bed, holding mom's hand, and I knew they had been praying as well. They looked up at me expectantly as I walked in.

I took a deep breath, and said, "God says that just because I'm a nurse doesn't mean I'm not still a human, and trusting Him means trusting you to decide what's best for you."

Mom smiled, knowingly. "That can't be easy for you, Allison," she said, softly.

"No," I sighed. "But if it was easy, it wouldn't be faith."

Dad nodded in agreement. "We were just discussing that, too," he said. "We decided that God can take care of her, and we're going to stay here."

I felt strangely relieved and terrified at the same time. The decision was no longer on my shoulders, but we had just eliminated our safety net. This trust thing wasn't for the faint of heart.

"Well, here's to trusting God," I said. I felt like I should 'cheers' to that, but I didn't have anything in my hand.

"Look at that!" Rhonda cried out from the desk. A moment later, she came bursting into the room. "You converted!" she practically screamed.

I looked up at the monitor, and sure enough- there was the most beautiful normal sinus rhythm I had ever seen. Mom and dad both looked at it too, a little perplexed about what we were seeing.

"Oh, look, it's only 76," mom commented. "And they all look the same now."

"Your heart went back in to a normal rhythm," I explained. "That's what we've been waiting for." My voice cracked on the last word and I felt tears prick my eyes. They were tears of joy, but I couldn't believe I was about to cry over this. I hadn't realized how scared I was.

"I have to call Dr. Lytle!" Rhonda exclaimed, and rushed back out to the desk. It warmed my heart that she was so excited that my mom was doing better. Some nurses are just doing the work that's necessary, but good nurses really care about how the patients do.

"So, I'm better?" mom asked, still a little unsure of what had happened.

"Mostly," I replied, not wanting to be a negative nancy, but I had to be honest. "There's always a chance you could go back into a-fib, so we have to wait a few hours to make sure you stay in sinus rhythm. And, obviously, you still have a blood clot in your lung that needs to dissolve. But this is a huge step in the right direction."

Rhonda came bustling back in to the room. "Dr. Lytle will be here in about ten minutes," she informed us, still smiling. Then she paused and cocked her head at mom. "Did you ever get lunch?" she asked her.

"Well, I wasn't really hungry," mom downplayed it. "I could eat something, though."

"I'm so sorry!" Rhonda cried. "I completely forgot! I'm not used to having to order trays. I'll call the kitchen right away."

I hadn't realized mom didn't eat, even when dad and I went for lunch. Funny how I felt like she was all I had thought about today, but obviously I wasn't paying that much attention. Of course, I didn't have the 'mom' factor that made me worry about other people and whether they had eaten or not.

My grandma was really obsessed with people eating. Any time I visited her, she was trying to feed me something every hour or so. Finally, I would take the food just to appease her, but then an hour later, she was convinced I must be hungry again. I always left there stuffed to the gills.

Dr. Lytle came in while we were waiting for lunch, a big grin plastered on his face. "Betty, you look fantastic!" he said, enthusiastically. "Best-looking gal I've seen all day, as a matter of fact."

"Thank you," mom said, chuckling, "but I don't think you thought that a few hours ago."

"No, I sure didn't," he agreed. "You have given me a run for my money today."

"Well, you came through with flying colors," mom assured him.

"I had some help," he reminded her, glancing toward me. I tried to act nonchalant, like it was no big deal. I was bad at accepting praise, I felt awkward and never knew what to say.

"We will wait a few hours to make sure your heart stays in this normal rhythm, and we'll start you on the oral version of this drug, just to be safe," he explained to mom. "I want to keep you in here one more night, just to have you on the monitor, mostly for my peace of mind."

"Ok," mom agreed. Rhonda came in with the lunch tray, which smelled like it was the same lasagna that dad and I had eaten. I suddenly felt hungry again, just smelling the food. I sure didn't need to eat lunch twice, especially since my day's activities had consisted of sitting and then sitting some more.

"I'll leave you to your lunch," Dr. Lytle said. "I'll call Dr. Boding and update him. Hopefully, we won't need his services anymore."

Dr. Lytle went back out to the desk and Rhonda arranged the tray on the bedside table and moved it over the bed so mom could eat. My stomach actually growled at the sight of food. Maybe stress burned lots of calories.

"I'm going to go stretch my legs for a bit," I said. I didn't want to sit here and watch my mom eat, and I needed to move around a little.

I wandered down the now-familiar halls, past the surgical waiting room and down to the ER. The waiting room had several people in it as I walked by. Now that the snow had stopped, people could get out and about again.

I skipped the gift shop, since I knew there would be sweet treats to tempt me. I wandered down the medical unit hallway, and noticed Lori sitting at the desk, doing something on her phone. I felt a flash of anger jolt through me. How could she just sit there? Her laziness and inattention to my mom had started this whole thing! If she just would have gotten off her fat butt and put my mom's SCDs on, we could have skipped this whole horrible situation. Did she even care? She could have killed my mom! It obviously hadn't changed her attitude about work. Didn't she realize how important her job was?

I stood there, burning in anger and frustration for a minute. I kind of wanted to go confront her about all of this, and I had about decided I was going to, when a thought flittered through my head- '*All things work together for good.*' All of this was part of God's plan, even though I couldn't understand why He did it. But I didn't want to just accept it, I still wanted to be mad at Lori. I wasn't so great at forgiving, and I was terrible at forgetting. But I was a pro at holding a grudge.

Karen walked around the corner at the end of the hall just then, and saw Lori sitting there, and me standing past her in the hall. She immediately realized what was going on, and started walking towards us.

"How are your patients doing, Lori?" she asked, bluntly. Lori jumped to her feet and tried to hide her phone by her side when she heard Karen's voice.

"Oh, um, good," she stammered. "I was just going to check on them."

"I figured you were," Karen said, pointedly. Lori scurried into the closest patient room, her cell phone still clutched in her hand. Karen walked down the hall to me.

"I know what you're thinking," she said to me. "I would be thinking the same thing."

"This whole thing could have been avoided," I said, angrily. "It's her fault and she doesn't even care!"

I didn't mean to sound like a whiny five-year-old, but it came out that way. I felt a little embarrassed, I was supposed to be a professional.

"I can't make her care," Karen said, "but we've had a long talk about her nursing care, and we're watching her closely. She knows she's on thin ice. She still plays on her phone, as you can see, but her call lights get answered pronto. And all her patients have their SCDs on!"

At least they were trying to improve her nursing care. Honestly, I had a coworker who was on his phone all the time, and I wondered how much stuff he missed because he was lazy and didn't care. There were always going to be bad nurses in this world.

"C'mon, I'll buy you a coffee and a snack," Karen said, gesturing down the hallway. As we walked away, I felt my anger fading. Being mad at Lori wasn't going to help anyone, and it was going to make me callous and bitter.

"We can't fix the bad nurses," Karen said, echoing my thoughts. "We can only make sure that we aren't one of them."

There was the life lesson for the day. Learned the hard way, as usual.

Chapter Sixteen

After our coffee break, Karen walked back to mom's room with me, just to check on her and say 'hi'. I felt a lot better after chatting with her. And I avoided the cookie and opted for a dish of Waldorf salad instead. Got some fruit and veggies and healthy nuts. And Cool Whip, but that was the part that made it taste good!

Mom was sitting up in the bed, and she was wearing the nasal oxygen tubing instead of the mask. Her cardiac monitor still showed sinus rhythm, which made me very happy. The longer she stayed in a normal rhythm, the less chance she would go back into a-fib.

"Karen, it's so good to see you!" mom said brightly. She was sounding more like her usual self.

"Betty, you look great, all things considered," Karen replied, smiling. "You are a tough lady."

"I don't know about that," mom said, chuckling. "I've had some fantastic help here, that's for sure."

I was glad my mom could remember all the good nurses and doctors. We had only had one bad nurse, but I kept getting hung up on remembering her. I needed to be more like my mom.

Mom and Karen visited for a while, while dad relaxed in the recliner and I paced around the room, bored. I finally started wandering up and down the hallway because the room was so small, I was getting dizzy.

"Need another book to read?" Rhonda asked me.

"No, I haven't finished the first one," I admitted. "I'm just not used to sitting around so much. I have some nervous energy to burn off and no way to do it."

"I can understand that," she replied. "Some days I wish there was a treadmill in here just so I could keep myself awake. I don't know how the night shift girls do it."

A treadmill would be great right now. I would be a lot less antsy after I ran a few miles. Of course, I wasn't in running shoes, and jeans weren't going to be that comfortable after the first half mile. I sighed and continued my pacing.

"Hey, I wanted to ask you about the telemedicine thing," Rhonda spoke up. I stopped at the desk to talk to her.

"How did you learn about that?" she asked. "It's really amazing, and if anybody could use it, it's us."

"There's a doctor at my work that is big into it," I told her. "He's always talking about it and how it's the future of rural medicine. To be honest, most of the time I sort of tune him out. I mean, he is *always* talking about it. But I must have listened enough to pick up the basics, and right now, I'm really glad I did!"

"For sure," she replied, emphatically. "I think we'll be using that again around here."

I got a little thrill of satisfaction at knowing I had impacted healthcare that way. That was what we were always hoping to do in this field, to make a difference in someone's health. It made me happy to know that someone down the road might benefit from what I had showed them today.

"How do you like working ER?" she asked me.

"I love it," I replied, automatically. "It's something different every day. Although some days are better than others," I added, smiling wryly.

"I've never worked ER," Rhonda said. "I just couldn't handle all the blood and gore."

I never knew what to say to that. Most of my shifts didn't involve any blood and gore. Some of my shifts involved abdominal pain and sore throats and people who just couldn't get a doctor's appointment. Some of my shifts involved whiny people who really didn't need to be in the ER at all. Those ones were harder for me to handle than the trauma patients. I had a hard time being patient with people who were just abusing the system.

"Well, it takes all kinds," I replied. "I don't know if I could do this job. There's a lot to know."

"True," Rhonda agreed. "Not as much here, we don't have anything too critical."

"My dad had open heart surgery in Springfield earlier this year," I told her. "Those nurses had some serious responsibility."

“Yeah,” Rhonda said wistfully. “I still miss it some days.”

I remembered her telling me that she had worked a cardiac unit before she moved here. Her move here probably hadn’t been her idea, since it was her husband’s family business. I wondered how it would feel to spend years building a career and then just have to walk away from it.

Of course, there was always an ER, so no matter where I lived, I could still work in my field. But some ERs had to be a lot more boring than others.

“At least you get to miss out on the drunks,” I said, chuckling.

“True. Although sometimes we have to watch an overdose patient until they come back around,” she replied. “They usually just sleep though. Except one girl we had- she had taken a bunch of her ADHD meds. I don’t know what she was trying to accomplish, but she whacked out. She kept hallucinating and seeing all kinds of creepy crawly things in the room. Spiders and snakes and giant bugs, and she would freak out! Screaming and swinging and climbing out of the bed. She even punched a nurse who was trying to calm her down. We had to put her in four-point restraints for a little while. It was horrible.” She shuddered at the memory.

Four-point restraints were serious business, and we only used them when we had absolutely no other choice. I didn’t like them either- they seemed so brutal- but I had been in situations where they were unavoidable. Meth users were the most common ones I saw that were just uncontrollable and violent. I had dodged a few punches myself, and one of my coworkers had been choked.

"It sounds horrible," I agreed with her. Nurses have some pretty interesting stories to tell. At the time they're happening, though, interesting isn't the word to describe them.

Karen came back out of mom's room and walked over to the desk to talk to Rhonda. I headed back into mom's room so I wouldn't be eavesdropping on their conversation.

"When do you plan on heading home?" mom asked me. She must be feeling well enough that she thought it was safe for me to leave.

"I was waiting to see how the roads were," I replied. "Shelby wants to come over when I leave, just so someone is here."

"Oh, she doesn't need to do that," mom protested. "You girls worry too much about me."

Honestly, I worried less about mom if one of us was with her. She could downplay her symptoms over the phone, but I knew Shelby would let me know pronto if something seemed out of the ordinary.

"That was the plan from the beginning," I reminded her. "The weather just changed the time for when I left and she arrived."

The road would probably open today, but I didn't want to be one of the first people back out on it. I had all-wheel drive in my car, but Shelby didn't in hers. By tomorrow, the road would be a little better, I figured. We would let all the people with four-wheel drive wear the snow and ice off.

I decided to call Shelby and see what she thought, as long as we were talking about it. I pulled out my phone and hit her name.

"Hey, 'Lis," she answered. She had probably just finished her lunch shift at Joe's. "How's mom?"

We had at least progressed to getting a 'hello' before asking about mom.

"Good," I told her. "She's still in a normal rhythm and she's off the oxygen mask and just on regular oxygen now. She feels better too, and she ate almost all of her lunch."

"Awesome!" Shelby said, excitedly.

"We were talking about when I would go home and you would come over," I went on.

"Is the road open?" she asked.

"No, but they were planning on opening it soon," I replied. "I would rather wait until tomorrow to drive it, though."

"Good idea," Shelby agreed. "Jamie at work said she would cover my shifts whenever I needed her to, so I can come over tomorrow. I just need someone to watch Snickers."

There was a long pause, and I knew Shelby wanted me to volunteer to take her. I really hated watching Snickers because, well, she was annoying. And spoiled. I usually tried to have a good excuse, but I was stymied this time. I didn't go back to work until Monday, so I couldn't use that.

"You could bring her with you and then she could play with Lady," I suggested. Mom glared at me. She didn't care for Snickers, either, and I don't know if Lady really liked having her around. Lady was sort of past the part of her life where she wanted to run around and play, she liked laying on her soft bed and getting petted. I was being a horrible sister and daughter, I realized.

"I'll take her," I sighed. I wasn't going to pretend to be happy about it, but I would at least do it.

"Great!" Shelby said. "She loves you!" Snickers did seem to love me, for some odd reason. I wasn't very nice to her, but she seemed oblivious to the fact that I didn't like her. So much for dogs being smart and perceptive. Snickers was the exception to that rule.

"Let's plan for tomorrow," I said. "I'll call you again when the road opens."

"Ok," Shelby replied. "Can I talk to mom?"

I handed mom the phone and sat there in silence, pouting that I had to take my sister's stupid, spoiled pug. I always got roped into watching her. I wondered if this trend would continue if Shelby had kids. I might be the perpetual dog/babysitter. Then I would have two things drooling on me, and I would have to clean up the poop for both of them.

I decided to escape into the book again for a while. It would take my mind off things, at least. I picked up the novel off the side table and searched for where I had left off. I had forgotten to stick a book mark in, and so much had happened since I stopped reading, it took a few minutes before I remembered enough about the story to figure out where I had stopped reading. I was stuck on the hard chair, but I didn't want to go to the waiting room until mom was done with my phone. I told myself I needed to have it close by to keep in touch with family, but truthfully, I wanted to have it in case Jake texted again. Not so much that I would see the text right away, but so my mom didn't pick up the phone and see it. I didn't want to be answering a lot of questions about this guy and why he was texting me.

Mom finished up with Shelby about the time my right butt cheek went numb, so I took my phone and excused myself to the waiting room. I still had the place to myself, so I stretched out on the couch and let my mind wander off into someone else's life for a while.

I woke up with a start, a creepy feeling jolting through me. I looked up and saw a man standing in the door, staring at me. He was wearing a hospital nametag that said 'Housekeeping', and a work uniform that hung loosely on his bony frame. He had shaggy, black hair and intense dark eyes, and he just stood there in eerie silence, drilling through me with his dark eyes. I actually felt frightened, even though he was shorter than I was and scrawny enough I could probably take him.

"I need to clean in here," he finally said, in a flat voice. I scrambled to my feet and grabbed the book that had fallen to the floor.

"I'll get out of your way," I said hastily and started for the door. He didn't move, however, so I couldn't really get around him.

"You can stay while I clean," he said. Right.

"No, I need to go see my mom," I said. "Excuse me." I gestured toward the doorway, to indicate that I needed to get out. He stepped back about six inches, leaving just a small space for me to get through. This guy was making my skin crawl. I couldn't really get through that space without having to touch him, but I was too creeped out to care. I rushed through the small space, bumping him enough that he lost his balance and had to take a step back. I smacked my other shoulder on the door jam, trying unsuccessfully to avoid him. I hurried down the hall to the ICU and I could feel him watching me.

I got through the door and breathed a sigh of relief. I was rubbing my shoulder where I had hit it as I walked past the desk.

"Are you ok?" Rhonda asked.

"I bumped my shoulder on the door jam," I said. "The housekeeping guy was standing in the doorway and I couldn't get through."

"Ah, that must have been Lance," she said. "He's done that to me before."

"He's creepy," I blurted out, before I could stop myself. Rhonda chuckled at that.

"Yes, he is. He's never actually done anything wrong enough that they can write him up, but he's just weird. He looks like he could easily snap and start stabbing people."

"He was watching me sleep," I told her. I shivered as I said it.

"Ick! I'm so sorry," Rhonda sympathized. "He only works until 4:30, so he'll be gone soon."

I was relieved to hear that. Then another thought occurred to me.

"Does he come in here to clean next?" I asked.

"I'll tell him he doesn't need to," Rhonda assured me. "We will close again tomorrow and he can clean then. It's not like we've gotten the place dirty. We've only been here 12 hours."

I was startled to realize that she was right- we had only been in the ICU for twelve hours. It felt like a week with everything that had happened.

I headed back in to mom's room. Dad looked up as I walked in and said, "They opened the road, but they're saying no unnecessary travel right now."

"We're going to wait until tomorrow," I told him.

"Good idea," he said. "Road will be better then."

"I kind of want to stay the night anyway," I confessed. "Just to be sure, I guess."

Dad smiled knowingly. "Figured you might."

I really needed to get out of this hospital for a little bit. I was restless and bored, and now Lance was creeping me out.

"Hey dad, how about if I go home and shovel off the walks?" I offered. "I can let Lady out and then come back a little later."

"Gettin' a little antsy, are you?" he said, smiling. He wasn't one to turn down a snow shoveling offer, and he readily handed me the truck keys. Now I had to get back out of the hospital without running into Lance. I grabbed my coat and gloves, checked that I had my cell phone and told them to call me if anything happened.

I said good-bye to Rhonda and walked quickly down the hall toward the front door. I wanted to look around for Lance as I walked, but I kept my eyes glued straight forward. That way, if I did pass him, I could pretend I didn't see him and just keep going. Luckily, I made it out without any more creepy encounters.

I started the truck and then brushed off the snow while the truck warmed up. I made sure to clear all the windows really well, to make sure I could see. Then I had to brush off the snow that had gotten all over the front of me during the process.

I climbed in the cab and it was still cold in there. I turned on the defrost but it was only cold air, so I sat impatiently waiting for it to get warm. The inside of the windows was starting to fog over from my breath, even though I was trying very carefully to breathe through my nose.

The windshield finally cleared enough that I could safely drive and I headed out of the parking lot. It was still cloudy but getting lighter and the streets were plowed. The steam from the hot springs pool billowed up in stark white clouds against the gray-white background of the sky. I drove home and parked in the garage so I could shovel the driveway. Dad had a snowblower that he used on the driveway and long sidewalk, but I figured the exercise would do me some good.

Lady was excited to see me and I petted her for a long time after she had emptied her bladder. We hadn't meant to be gone for that long, but we weren't really thinking about it when we left at 4 o'clock this morning.

I got the shovel and started from the front door out. I cleaned the steps thoroughly, I knew my mom was always afraid of slipping on them. Of course, she probably wouldn't be going up and down the steps for a while with her knee, but safe steps were always a good idea. I started down the front sidewalk, thankful that it was a fairly light snow. In the spring, the snow could get wet and really heavy. This wasn't too difficult to shovel.

I did the sidewalks and then I stopped and took a breather for a while. Shoveling snow was hard work. That was why we always got a couple guys in every winter who had a heart attack while they were shoveling snow. My heart was healthy, but it was sure pounding away right now. My hands and feet were cold, but I was starting to break a sweat.

I started back up with the driveway, reminding myself that I needed the exercise and this would work off some stress. Plus, I wasn't totally sure how to run the snowblower, so I was stuck with the shovel.

I finally finished the driveway, with a couple more breaks to catch my breath. I felt accomplished, looking at the cleared concrete. It was good to have something to actually do, after three days of sitting around.

I went inside and peeled off my coat and gloves. Lady looked up at me curiously and then went back to her nap. My face was red from the cold and my nose was running. I felt better, but I looked terrible, I'm sure.

Once I had blown my nose and gotten a drink, I wandered over to pet Lady again. I wasn't very excited to go back to the hospital and sit around, so I was trying to find excuses not to go back yet. We hadn't been here much this week, so there wasn't really laundry or dishes to do. I sat there, scratching Lady's ears absently, trying to kill time.

I finally sighed and stood up. I couldn't think of anything else to do, so I decided I might as well head back. I climbed into the truck and backed out of the garage. Dad's truck was a lot bigger than my car and it felt a little weird driving it. I probably looked like a teenage driver, I was driving slow and taking wide turns.

It was already getting dark when I got back to the hospital. I realized I was getting hungry and it was almost suppertime. Dad and I would have to decide what to do for dinner. I couldn't wait to be back home with my kitchen and fridge. I wasn't going to eat out for a month.

Mom still looked great and dad looked bored. Being the family member of a hospital patient was frustrating-stressful and monotonous all at once. I would be very glad when we were out of here, and I hoped we weren't back in a hospital for a very long time.

Mom, as usual, was worried about everyone eating, so she brought up the subject of supper right away. Dad agreed that he could eat something, so we decided to head to the grocery store and pick something up from their deli. I could get some fruit to eat as well. Rhonda was ordering mom's supper tray, so we could grab our food and come back to eat with her. Although it would be the oddest family dinner we had ever had.

After we got done eating, we sat around and chatted for awhile. I was avoiding the topic of going home, but I was fairly certain Shelby and I would be trading spots tomorrow. I was homesick but nervous about leaving, just the same. I had to trust Shelby to watch out for mom, and she had done a great job standing up for dad when he needed someone in his corner. I didn't have any reason to doubt her. Mom was looking much better, so I was probably worrying for no reason. As usual.

I hugged mom good night and then stepped out in the hall while my dad said good-bye to her. It felt weird to stand there and watch my parents canoodle. They were a loving couple, and I'm sure this was hard for them to be apart this much. Well, in a couple days, things would go back to mostly normal.

We said good night to Rhonda and thanked her for everything. It was only fifteen minutes until her relief showed up, it was Gina again tonight. I hoped she had gotten a good sleep today, because it was going to be a long, boring night for her.

"Wow, the driveway looks good," dad commented as we pulled in. "Did you use the snowblower?"

"No, I wasn't sure how to run it," I replied. "Besides, I needed the exercise."

"Better you than me," dad chuckled. We walked in the house and Lady came rushing over to meet us. She greeted each of us, and then looked past us, perplexed. She was still looking for mom.

"It's ok, girl, she'll be home in a couple days," I assured her. Of course, she had no idea what I was saying, but I felt better at least trying to comfort her.

I checked my phone as I was relaxing on the couch. I had a missed call from work, which made me curious. There was a voicemail, so I listened to it. It was my co-worker, Linda.

'Jake was just in and mentioned your mom was having complications. Hope she's doing better and if you have to stay longer, let me know and I can cover your shifts for you."

That was so sweet of her to be worried about me and my mom. I had some great co-workers, that was for sure. Of course, Linda was probably wondering why Jake knew about the details of my family's life, and if that meant there was something going on between us. Linda wanted me to get together with Jake, so she was probably hoping that a romance was brewing.

I sent a quick text to Shelby and Andrew and let them know mom was still doing great and we had gone home for the night. I would call Shelby in the morning about the driving plan after I saw the road report. I scrolled through Facebook to see what was going on in everyone else's world. Nothing too exciting but it was a nice distraction for awhile. I couldn't decide if I was tired or just bored, but I finally decided to go to sleep.

The next morning, my shoulders yelled at me as soon as I tried to get out of bed. Guess I got a good workout with the snow shovel! I gingerly stretched out and tried to loosen my muscles up. Once I could finally get dressed, I headed out to the kitchen. Dad had the weather channel on and was watching for the road report.

I poured a cup of coffee and made a piece of toast for breakfast. I had already decided in my head I was going home today, so I hoped the weather cooperated. I got pretty irritated when things didn't go according to my plan. Which meant I got irritated a lot.

"Looks like it's pretty clear," dad commented.

"Ok, I'll call Shelby," I said, reaching for my phone. I noticed the blinking light telling me I had a text message. Who was up this early?

'Just went out Hwy 24 on a call. Road is nice and dry. Drive safe!' the message from Jake read. It sure was handy to have a friend on the fire department sometimes.

I dialed Shelby, who didn't answer until the fifth ring. As usual.

"'llo," she mumbled. I guess I could have waited to call her later, but she needed to be awake anyway, so she could pack a bag and get headed down the road.

"Morning, sunshine!" I chirped, mirroring our mom. I was greeted with an incredibly long stretch of silence.

"Morning," Shelby finally muttered. "Is everything ok?"

"Yes, and the road is open and dry, so we need to switch spots," I told her.

"Right now?!" she snapped back.

"Um, well, soon," I hedged. I didn't want to sit around all day again. Or even half of the day. I was anxious to get home, now that mom was doing so well.

Shelby sighed. "I'll text you when I leave," she finally said. "Later."

I hung up and told dad that Shelby would be headed out in a while. Probably more than an hour from now, because Shelby didn't move quickly in the morning. I could be ready to go in ten minutes flat, but I didn't have much for a beauty routine.

I packed my bags and loaded them in my car. Dad and I would drive separately to the hospital and I would just leave from there when Shelby arrived. I had to brush all the snow off my car and scrape the windshield. I hadn't driven it since Sunday.

We walked through the doors into the ICU, and I was so lost in my thoughts, I didn't notice anything different. The first thing I did notice was Lance, standing in the doorway of mom's room, with his housekeeping cart sitting in the hallway. A shiver ran down my spine, remembering how creepy he had been yesterday. I didn't want him anywhere near my mom. I took a quick couple steps toward her room and then realized it was empty. The bed had all the linens stripped off of it and Lance was mopping the floor. I whirled back around to the nurses' station and saw that it was empty as well.

"Where's my mom?!" I cried out, panicked, to no one in particular.

"She moved out," Lance answered flatly. I stared at him, perplexed. Moved out to where? The road was open, did they transfer her in the middle of the night and not call us? My mind was racing and my heart was too.

"Oh good, you're here," I heard Karen's voice say, cheerily. I spun around and looked at her, still wondering what was going on.

"Where's mom?" I asked, a touch of panic creeping into my voice. Karen looked startled.

"She transferred back out to the medical floor just now," she said. "Didn't Lance tell you?"

"Not exactly," I said, shaking and willing my heart to slow back down. Karen scowled past me at Lance, and then shook her head in frustration.

"I'm so sorry," she apologized profusely. "We transferred her back out to the medical floor at the end of night shift, so we wouldn't have to bring in the day nurse for one hour and then send her home. She's doing great, and Dr. Lytle has already been around to see her this morning."

I was nodding as she talked, trying to stay focused on her words. My moment of panic was silly, and I was a little embarrassed about it, but for some reason, my mind had jumped to the worst possible conclusion when my mom's bed was empty.

"I'll walk you to her room," Karen offered, looking at me sympathetically. "I'm really sorry about this."

"I don't know why I'm so jumpy," I admitted to her as we walked back down the hall. "Obviously, Gina would have called if anything was wrong."

"Sometimes, emotion overrides common sense," Karen said. "Remember me telling you how horrible I was to my mom's nurses? I knew better, but somehow, that didn't stop me. I guess we are human, after all," she laughed.

We were at the door of room 126, and Karen pointed in to the room. Dad and I walked in and saw mom, sitting up in the recliner. She looked so beautiful, I wanted to cry. She still had the oxygen on, but otherwise, she looked like my mom again. I walked over and gave her a hug, trying to blink away the tears before she could see them.

Maybe this whole ordeal had just worn me down. I wasn't normally an emotional, teary person. Maybe the seriousness of what had happened was finally catching up to me. Maybe I was tired and just needed more coffee.

But most likely, I had realized how close I came to losing my mom.

Chapter Seventeen

Shelby finally arrived about 10 o'clock, looking adorable, as always. I knew her hair fell in those long ringlets naturally, so that wasn't what took her so long to get ready. I never had figured out what she had to do in the morning, she always looked gorgeous, any time of day. Mom and dad were both happy to see her, and we sat around and chatted for a bit. It would only take me an hour to drive home, so I wasn't in a huge rush. Once I got back to Brighton, I was in charge of Snickers, and I wasn't super excited about that.

"Oh, by the way, I just left Snickers at your house," Shelby mentioned nonchalantly, after she had been there forty-five minutes.

"She's in my house?" I cried. I thought she had left her in her apartment and I would have to go get her. Instead, she was happily chewing up my stuff while I was just sitting here.

"Well, I thought it would be easier for you," Shelby sniffed. "I was trying to save you some trouble."

Fail. Leaving Snickers alone in my house for three hours did not save me trouble at all. I hastily said good-bye to mom and dad, hugged them both extra tight and told them I would call when I got home. I hopped in the car and headed down the road.

Driving always gave me lots of time to think, which was good some days and bad other days. Today was a good day, I had a lot to mull over from the last week, but nothing to worry about. Well, except my furniture. But my mom was doing great, everything had worked out just fine and in a couple days she would be home. I had the weekend to relax and get ready to go back to work. And, apparently, I didn't even have to shovel snow when I got home.

That thought got my mind to wandering and wondering about Jake. Had he really shoveled my sidewalk? How would I find out? And what should I say? I didn't want to come right out and ask him, what if he hadn't done it? Then he might wonder why I thought he would shovel my walk. I didn't know who else would have done it. It could have been the neighbor, or someone from church. Several people knew I was going to be out of town for my mom's surgery, and maybe someone was just being nice.

I pulled up to my house, feeling suddenly tired but very glad to be home. Sure enough, my sidewalk was meticulously groomed, even my front porch steps were cleared off. I was grateful, even if I didn't know who had done it.

I grabbed my bags and headed inside to see what damage Snickers had done. She came barreling at me as soon as she heard the door open, snorting and snuffling and jumping up on me. I had a bag in each hand, so I couldn't even push her back down. I was trying to walk to my bedroom to set the bags down, but Snickers kept jumping on me and trying to trip me. I accidently stepped on her more than once, but she still didn't get out of the way. That dog was not the brightest bulb.

I finally got my bags set down and petted Snickers enough to get her to calm down. I started walking around my house, surveying for damage. I didn't see anything too out of place. She had chewed up a magazine and there were muddy little paw prints on the refrigerator door.

I called Shelby's cell phone to tell her I had made it home. She said mom walked to the bathroom and back, and was in the chair, waiting for lunch. That news was delightfully boring and exactly what I wanted to hear.

I unpacked my bags and threw in a load of laundry. I needed to hit the grocery store, I had deliberately left an empty fridge on Sunday. I snagged a granola bar and munched on it while I put stuff away. Sometimes, I wondered what they put in them that made them safe to keep on a shelf for a year and still eat. Then I decided I probably didn't want to know.

I got everything put away and then stretched out on top of my bed, relishing being back home again. My place wasn't that big or nice, but it was my home and I had missed it. I was relaxing and contemplating a nap when my phone buzzed.

'*Did you make it home ok?*' Jake wanted to know. It was sweet that he was worried about me.

'*Yep. Safe and sound. It's good to be home.*' I replied.

'How did your house look?' he asked, with a smiley face. I guess we knew who had shoveled my walk.

'Great! Some wonderful person shoveled all my snow. Which was very, very nice of them to do,' I wrote back.

'He takes cookies as a thank you, if you were so inclined,' Jake informed me. It was funny how he was so concerned with working out, but still indulged in sweet treats whenever he got the chance.

'I'll see if I can't pick up some supplies at the store. This weather is made for baking!'

Of course, I didn't know when I was going to see Jake next, and there wasn't much point in baking cookies and just having them sit around my house. I would eat them, and I did not need to eat cookies.

'Let me know when they're done and I'll stop over.' Jake solved that dilemma for me. Which meant I also needed to shower and do something with my hair before I finished the cookies.

I got up to start a grocery list before I fell asleep on top of the bed. I looked through the fridge and cupboards, writing down what I needed. Snickers saw me opening the fridge and came waddling over to see if she could beg some treats, then waddled back to her bed when she realized she wasn't getting anything.

The grocery store was busy, but I got through there quickly. I got home, put the groceries away, set some butter out in a mixing bowl to soften and jumped in the shower. I blow-dried my hair with a round brush and some shine serum, going for the natural and glossy look. I basically wanted it to look like it hadn't required any work at all, which took a lot of work.

Once my hair was satisfactory, I mixed up the cookie dough while the oven heated. I snitched a couple bites of dough while I was putting it on the cookie sheet, as always.

'Going in the oven now,' I sent a message to Jake. My stomach was fluttery at the thought of Jake coming over to my house, but I was trying to keep a cool exterior. Making cookies was just a way to say 'thank you' for shoveling all my snow. It would be rude of me not to show my appreciation for all his hard work.

I took the first pan out and slid the second pan in. I was savoring the aroma of fresh-baked cookies when a knock at the front door startled me. I walked to the door, opened it and was surprised to see Jake standing there.

"Are they done yet?" he asked earnestly, looking like a little kid. I laughed.

"The first pan just came out," I said, as I stood back so he could come inside. He walked in, pulling off his jacket, and headed straight for the kitchen. I followed him in there, and he was standing at the counter, staring at the cookies still on the pan.

"Those are beautiful," he said, dramatically. "Almost too beautiful to eat."

I arched my eyebrow at him.

"Just kidding! Where's the scooper thing?" he asked. I pulled a spatula out of the drawer and handed it to him.

"They might not be cool enough to eat yet," I started to warn him, but he already had one scooped up and shoved half of it in his mouth.

"Mmm-hmm," he mumbled in appreciation around the mouthful of cookie. He had a drop of melted chocolate chip on his chin and another one smeared on his cheek. He didn't seem to care, he scooped up another cookie and ate it with gusto.

I just giggled as I watched him devour the cookies like he was starving. I have to admit, eating chocolate chip cookies still warm and gooey out of the oven is one of life's great pleasures. Watching Jake eat chocolate chip cookies in my kitchen was just about as good.

He finally stopped after the fourth one and took a look around. "Do you have any milk?" he asked.

I got a glass and poured him some milk, and he chugged half of it in two swallows. Apparently, firemen are used to eating fast. Kind of like nurses- some days you only had a few minutes to eat, there was no time to waste on chewing and tasting stuff.

The timer chirped and I took the second pan of cookies out. I reached for the bowl to put the rest of the dough on a sheet and in the oven. Jake saw the bowl of cookie dough and his eyes lit up all over again.

"Cookie dough! Can I eat it?" he asked excitedly.

"Sure," I said, handing him the bowl. It saved me the trouble of baking it. He leaned back against the counter as he picked out wads of dough and ate them.

"How's mom and everyone?" he asked around bites of dough.

"Mom is great," I replied. "She moved back out to the medical floor this morning and will probably go home tomorrow or Sunday. Dad is good, bored from sitting in a hospital all day. Shelby is there with them now, just in case. Which means I have Snickers."

As if on cue, Snickers waddled into the kitchen and stood at Jake's feet, begging for food. He looked down at her, then shrugged and went back to eating. I guess her puppy dog eyes didn't work on Jake- he wasn't sharing the cookie dough.

"When do you work again?" he asked.

"Monday," I replied. "So I have the weekend to catch up on everything. Including sleep. It's amazing how tiring it is to sit around all day."

"Yeah, I've been there," Jake said. "I think it's cause we aren't used to it." That sounded weird but it actually made sense.

"I work tomorrow and Monday," Jake informed me. "So I'll probably get to see you. We've been busy lately. Starting in with the snow shoveling heart attacks already."

"I shoveled my parents' whole driveway. I thought I might have a heart attack myself," I admitted. "But I needed something to do, I was going crazy just sitting there."

"Good thing you didn't have to shovel more when you got home, huh?" Jake asked, eyes twinkling.

I smiled warmly at him. In fact, I was feeling pretty warm all over, standing there with Jake, and I don't think it was because the oven was on.

"That was a very nice thing to do," I said. "I really appreciate it."

"Don't tell anyone I'm a nice guy, though," he warned me. "I have a reputation to maintain."

I giggled. Everyone knew Jake was a nice guy, but he was always joking that he was tough and mean.

"I have to get going," he sighed, scowling. "My mom needs help with something, and I promised her I would come right over."

"But then you stopped her for cookies?" I raised my eyebrows in feigned shock.

"See? Lying to my mom. How bad it that?" he replied. "But, in my defense, it was freshly baked chocolate chip cookies. Mom probably only had a meatloaf or something in the oven."

"You need to take these cookies with you," I said, firmly. "They cannot stay here." I grabbed a container from the cupboard and scooped the cookies in to it. They weren't completely cooled, so they were going to end up being one giant mash of cookie, but I was sure Jake would still eat them.

"There's just a little bit of cookie dough left," Jake said, innocently. "Should I leave it here?" He grinned at me wickedly.

I thought about acting virtuous but my sweet tooth won out. "I suppose," I said, reluctantly. "I could force myself to eat it."

"Are you at least going to bake it first?"

"Maybe," I replied, vaguely. "Or maybe I'll go green and save the electricity."

"Uh, your oven is still on," he reminded me with a smirk.

I sighed. "Busted. Well, I'll eat some dough and bake the rest. That's my plan."

"It's good to have a plan when it comes to cookie dough," Jake said. I agree.

"Ok, I really have to go," Jake said. Abruptly, he reached out and grabbed me, pulling me into his arms and squeezing me tight. "It's good to have you home," he said softly, resting his cheek on my head. He kept me wrapped in his strong arms for a glorious five seconds and then reluctantly loosened his grasp without completely letting go.

Wow. Maybe I should leave more often.

He finally released me all the way, now that I was tingling from head to toe. He shrugged into his jacket, grabbed his cookies, said a quick good-bye and headed out the door.

I realized after he left that I had been holding my breath, and slowly exhaled. I was suddenly very excited to go to work on Monday, and secretly hoping there were lots of ambulance calls. How wrong is that?!

Monday morning at 5:30, when the alarm went off, I was a little less excited about going to work. I had slept plenty over the weekend, so I should be all rested up. I just wasn't back in the swing of my usual routine.

I got out the door on time, even with having to scrape all my windows and wait for the car to warm up. It had been nice having dad do all that stuff for me, I had gotten a little spoiled. We hadn't had any more snow, so the roads were clear and I got to work just fine.

The morning started with a cup of coffee, as always. Monday mornings were usually pretty slow, so I could ease back into work mode. By 9 o'clock, I had one patient with nausea and vomiting and one patient with an abscess that needed drained. Dr. Wallace was eating breakfast and he wanted to finish that before we drained the abscess. Which was a good idea, because those procedures could kill your appetite.

I was standing at the desk when Dr. Raymond walked in the back door, carrying a stack of papers. I was excited to see him and tell him about our experience with telemedicine.

"Dr. Raymond," I called out, as I hurried down the hall toward him. "I wanted to talk to you."

He smiled in acknowledgement, but his stack of papers was starting to slide and he was hurrying toward the doctor office to set them down before they fell. He got to the desk just in time, and the papers landed in a pile.

"Yes, Allie," he said, breathlessly, turning toward me. "How are you?"

"I'm good," I said, out of habit. "My mom had knee surgery last week and she developed a DVT and then threw a PE. After that, she went into a-fib."

"And you're good?" he asked, eyebrows drawn together. Ok, that didn't come out right.

"Well, yes, I am now," I hastened to explain. "We were in Madison, that's where she lives, and they had this same snowstorm. So they couldn't transfer her out to Springfield, and the doctor there really didn't know what to do. I remembered what you had told me about telemedicine, so we went on the website and contacted a cardiologist. It was great! He even did an assessment of my mom over a video call. That was a little weird for her, but she finally got used to it.

"Anyway, he recommended a diltiazem drip and then checked back two hours later and she had converted back to sinus rhythm. It was great! Dr. Lytle was the surgeon there and he loved it. He was so concerned about mom and not being able to help her. I mean, he's a great doctor, but he's a surgeon in a small town, and he admitted that this wasn't something he ever had to deal with. The cardiologist- a Dr. Boding- was so good. I'm not sure what we would have done without him."

I had been rattling on a mile a minute, and I finally stopped to take a breath. Dr. Raymond was grinning so wide, I thought his face might crack.

"That's wonderful!" he exclaimed. "I didn't know if you were even listening half the time I was talking about it. But you were, and when you needed it, you had it. That's fantastic!"

I didn't admit to Dr. Raymond that half the time he was talking, I *wasn't* listening. More like three-fourths the time. In the end, I had heard enough of what he said to help my mom.

"So, how is your mom now?" he wanted to know.

"Great. Back on the medical floor, in sinus rhythm, and going home today. They kept her one extra night just to be safe."

"Did he have any trouble using it?" Dr. Raymond asked.

"No, he had a tablet that did the video call, and it was really easy to use. I left your name and number with him, I'm sure you'll be getting a call for more information," I told him.

"Wonderful!" he replied, still grinning. "This is what I've been telling you! The future of rural medicine!"

I had never seen Dr. Raymond look so enthused. He was normally a very serious and studious looking fellow. He looked ten years younger with his face lit up like that.

"Well, I just wanted to tell you about that," I said. "And to say 'thank you' for helping my mom, indirectly, at least."

"Helping people is the best part of this job," he said. I had to agree.

I went back to check on my patients, who were both doing fine. Dr. Wallace was finished with breakfast and was ready for the dirty work. I went in the room with him.

Stan Walkins had thought he had a spider bite on the inside of his upper arm. When it kept getting bigger and more painful, he thought it was just irritation from rubbing on his shirt. When the red, angry circle became the size of an orange, his wife insisted he come in.

Dr. Wallace numbed the area with lidocaine, being generous with the amount. Sometimes, I felt he was a little stingy with how much numbing he gave. But we both knew that with infected areas like this, the lidocaine wasn't as effective, so he gave plenty. Once it had had a few minutes to work, he scrubbed the area and reached for the scalpel.

Stan had been watching with interest up to that point, but this was where things got gross.

"You might not want to watch," I told him, gently.

"Heck, I've seen worse than that," he replied, dismissively. "I've gutted deer and neutered calves, so I'm used to blood and guts. Won't be a problem," he told me, boastfully.

Dr. Wallace shrugged and stuck the scalpel into the center of the hard, reddened lump. As expected, the pus inside came gushing out, mixed with a little blood. He soaked it up with some gauze pad and then pushed on the area to make sure all the fluid was out. I had been watching what he was doing, out of habit more than fascination. Stuff like this was gross, but I was used to it. I glanced at Stan to see what he thought.

Stan was staring intently at his arm, with an odd look on his face. And his face was mostly drained of any color. About then, his eyes rolled back in his head and his head flopped back on to the gurney. I guess Stan wasn't as tough as he thought.

Dr. Wallace had also noticed Stan's reaction to the events, and he snickered to himself. "The bigger they are, the harder they fall," he said, under his breath.

Stan didn't need to be awake for this, so we finished the procedure and let him 'sleep'. Once Dr. Wallace was finished, I touched Stan's arm and shook him gently to wake him up.

Stan sat up groggily and looked around, confused for a moment. Then he remembered where he was and looked a little embarrassed.

"I got a little lightheaded is all," he insisted. "I, uh, I didn't eat no breakfast."

"No biggie," I said lightly, hiding a smile. "We finished up without you." He smiled, sheepishly. I told him I would be back in a few minutes with discharge instructions. I was going to take my time getting him out the door, because I knew from personal experience that it takes about twenty minutes before you feel human again. I needed him recovered before he got in his truck to drive off.

I walked back out to the desk, where Dr. Wallace and I exchanged knowing smiles. I glanced up and saw that the ambulance crew was putting someone into the respiratory room, but it looked like they had the situation handled in there. My heart skipped a beat when I saw Jake's muscular shoulders straining against his t-shirt. Luckily, he was standing away from me as they lifted the patient, so he couldn't see me ogling him. Or turning red.

I looked back down at the chart in my hand, studying it intently without actually reading anything on it. The downside to seeing Jake at work was that I had to pretend like I wasn't excited to see Jake. Luckily, my coworker was Jesse today, and he didn't get too involved in my life, so I wouldn't have any prying questions to answer.

Jake and Kent finished settling their patient and walked back out to the desk. I prayed fervently that my face had returned to its usual color, and looked up with a smile.

"Hey guys, how's it going?" I asked casually, directing it at both of them.

"We're good, Allie," Kent answered, while Jake just smiled at me. "We're even better now that you're here."

"Glad I could brighten your day," I replied, glibly. Kent was always very friendly toward me. I wondered if Jake ever said anything about me as they were sitting around the station.

"How's your mom doing?" Kent asked. Apparently, Jake at least talked about my family. I filled Kent in on mom's status, trying not to look at Jake. He was fiddling with a vase of flowers that was sitting on the desk. It had been a 'thank you' from a patient's family, and it was a bit past its prime. Most of the flowers were wilted and turning brown, but no one had bothered to throw it away yet.

"Well, I'm glad she's doing better," Kent said. "Good thing you were there when she needed you!"

I nodded in agreement. I was very thankful I had been there for everything that happened.

Kent stepped away from the desk like he was going to head back out to the rig. Jake looked up from the flowers, and I saw he had picked out the few remaining alive blooms and had them clutched together in his hand.

"Here, Allie," he said, holding them out toward me with a smile. "I got you flowers."

The End

Acknowledgements

I have to thank God, first and foremost, for giving me the brain to be a nurse and an author, as well as a passion for both.

I want to thank my mother, Kit Fanning, for giving me a passion for reading and an affinity for big words.

Thank you to Dr. Barry Mangus and Wanda Hannebrink, RN, for their professional input on this novel.

Thank you to Kit Fanning and my grandma, Kay Gray, for the proofreading.

Thank you to all my friends and family who supported me in this venture, bought my first book, and repeatedly asked me when the next one was coming out.

About the Author

Stormy Fanning has been a nurse for over fifteen years and an avid reader since childhood. She enjoys spending time in the great outdoors and makes her home in Sheridan, WY.

This is the second in a series. The fictional town of Madison is loosely based on Thermopolis, WY, although any similarities to the hospital and its care are coincidental. As in the first book, the importance of good nursing care is emphasized, as it positively impacts the patient outcome.

Made in the USA
Monee, IL
05 November 2026

68006395R00198